D0755749

000002156066

EMERGENCY ADMISSIONS

Memoirs of an Ambulance Driver

KIT WHARTON

4th ESTATE · London

4th Estate
An imprint of HarperCollins*Publishers*
1 London Bridge Street
London SE1 9GF
www.4thEstate.co.uk

First published in Great Britain in 2017 by 4th Estate
This 4th Estate paperback edition published in 2018

1

DUDLEY LIBRARIES	
000002156066	
Askews & Holts	09-Apr-2018
	£8.99
2KF	

For Ren and Fin

CONTENTS

DISCLAIMER

This is a journal I've kept since joining an NHS emergency ambulance service trust somewhere in England in 2003. And an explanation of why I joined in the first place.

It's the best job in the world. I'm still learning. Often about people. If you even think you know them, you don't know them well enough. What did Robert Capa say? If your pictures aren't good enough, you're not close enough.

I should point out I'm not a doctor or nurse or even a paramedic. Pretty much the whole NHS is better qualified than I am. I've said to many a patient: no point asking me – thick as a whale sandwich – you might as well ask the cat. I just *take* you to see the right people. I should also point out I'm not a professional writer. If you're expecting Marcel Proust you might be disappointed. The journal is not endorsed by any ambulance service and no views expressed should be taken as those of one. Nothing should be taken as medical advice. All mistakes are my own. And some procedures and practices may have changed since I wrote about them.

Nothing has been invented or exaggerated – I wish some of it had, and actually I've toned some of it down – but names, locations, dates, sexes, medical conditions, characters and other details have been changed, disguised or amalgamated to protect anonymity.

One more caveat. A 'normal' job would be: called to a patient, say, fallen over. Patient is conscious or unconscious, and has no injuries/some injuries/lots of injuries. Patient is checked out and left at home or taken to hospital, where patient makes a good recovery/a partial recovery/unfortunately dies. The sort of job we do every day. Thousands of times a day.

The following are not normal jobs.

And you may need a strong stomach for a few of them…

1

JUST ANOTHER SHIFT...

All human life is here, as the *News of the World* used to say. On this shift, even more than usual.

Robert, Edward and Davina

It's the sunny evening of a bright spring day, but not in the mind of the next patient. We get a 999 call to Robert, in his fifties, with a long history of mental illness.

Robert is a tall thin man, with sunken eyes. He's hearing voices in his head, telling him to hurt himself, or someone else. He's tried to hurt himself in the past – and succeeded. You can see the scars all over his body.

Because of the nature of the job, the police come along and we meet them at the address. It's a pretty cottage, isolated down a track, with a lovely view over fields of corn and only the hum of the motorway to spoil things. But the garden tells you things are not right. There's an old sleeping bag in the middle of the grass, lots of other rubbish, and empty bottles and cans everywhere. No one's exactly been pruning the roses. Pity. Wouldn't mind living here myself.

But I wouldn't want what's going with it today.

We go in with the police to find a male lying in bed, bottles all over the floor and the room filthy. Dirty clothes and faeces everywhere. The patient's eyes stare into another world where you wouldn't want to go. There's an empty litre of off-brand gin by the bed – he's drunk it this morning – and a large kitchen knife. The WPC steps forward and removes it.

—We won't be needing that, will we?

She leaves us. I'm 'attending' this job, which means I deal with the patient. My crewmate stays outside with the police.

2

I talk to him gently for a bit just so he can get used to me and not feel threatened.

I ask whether he's happy to go to hospital.

—Yes.

—Super. Well let's get some trousers on, shall we? (Usually a good idea to keep it bright and breezy.)

—OK.

He gets up and crosses to the cupboard in the corner. Out of it – wordlessly – he pulls a bloody great machete, maybe three foot long, which he looks at and weighs in his hand as if he's buying it in a shop. No sign of any trousers.

Shit.

—I don't think we'll be needing that, will we, mate!

I say it loudly, so the police hear and, since it's all gone a bit pear-shaped, I back out of the room.

The coppers are outside in the corridor. I tell them what's happened.

—All right. Get outside.

From the front door we can hear the 'discussion' that follows.

—Put it down, Robert!

Nothing.

—Put it down!

More nothing.

—Put it down or we fucking spray you! Now!

The police carry pepper sprays and the like, but it's not good using them in a confined space like this.

My crewmate's called Valerie. Ten years younger than me, a lot prettier, but twenty years older when it comes to things like common sense. She has that weird and annoying

3

female gift, the ability to be right, about everything, all the time.

—We don't want to get involved in this. That stuff's horrible.

She drags me out.

Within a minute there are sounds of a scuffle and the handcuffed patient comes out with the two police either side of him. Under the anaesthetic of a litre of gin, Robert is unaffected, but the two coppers are suffering terribly, coughing and wheezing and spluttering, and the patient's holding them both up as they cling on to him like children.

We grab the patient and bundle him into the ambulance with a seatbelt on him, where he sits admiring the scene, while we put oxygen masks on the police who are sitting on the bonnet of their car and trying to breathe again.

It takes a good twenty minutes for the spray to wear off.

Then we take all three down to A&E.

Later in the shift.

Somewhere in England, not sure where. Don't really care, frankly. Busy shift – aren't they all? – but this one's a killer. Cold, foggy and damp. Nine in the evening. Exhausted and still three hours to go.

We're driving through the middle of nowhere.

We see about the tenth fox of the night. And a badger. Val thinks she's seen an owl, though she may be hallucinating. You can't do night shifts on the road without becoming interested in wildlife.

4

We get a 999 call to a male, late twenties, with abdominal pain. The address is a council flat in a block, quite respectable, a frightened-looking elderly couple in the front room. No male, late twenties.

Edward's their son. They tell us he's left and gone down the pub – even though he's barred and it's closed. Odd. He's an alcoholic and a frequent caller. Lots of 'previous' with us and the police. There's a warrant out for his arrest – for shoplifting or something.

Wow! How bad can he be? We look at their frightened faces and hazard a guess. Then down outside the pub we find out.

He's a wreck.

Filthy, stick-thin, with a grey pallor and sunken red eyes. Stinking of urine, vomit, sweat, you name it. Living rough and killing himself as fast as he can. Schizophrenic and alcoholic. He calls ambulances because whenever he gets sober enough to feel anything, his liver and pancreas – collapsing and inflamed through alcohol abuse – cause him agony. Then when he feels better, out of hospital he goes. It's difficult to know what will break the cycle, except the obvious. I think of the terrified look on his mother's gentle face.

At least he's not violent. As we get him on the ambulance the police turn up.

—Is it him?

—Yes. Do you know him?

—Oh yes. Where're you taking him? He normally goes to the local A&E.

—We'll take him to our A&E. Give his usual one a rest.

5

—OK. We'll come down and arrest him later.

In the ambulance he tells the policeman half-heartedly to fuck off then falls asleep – snoring and peeing himself – on the stretcher. The smell is bad. We set off. Halfway to hospital he wakes up and tries to focus.

—Who the fuck are you?

—Er, I'm the fucking ambulance man. You're in an ambulance.

—Where are we?

—On the way to D— — A&E.

—Don't want to fucking go there. I go to L— —!

—Well we're giving L— — a rest tonight, aren't we?

—No!

He gets out his phone – with difficulty – and dials 999.

—I want an ambulance.

—You're already in an ambulance! I shout, so the 999 call-taker can hear.

He continues to demand another ambulance, swearing into the phone, then hands it over.

—She wants to talk to you.

I press his phone to my ear.

—You've got a right twat there, the call-taker says cheerfully.

—Yes I know.

At hospital we unload him off into A&E. He lasts about two hours there, then wakes up and walks out. The police never show up.

—Bless, says Val.

He'll probably be back at his favourite hospital tomorrow. Can't help thinking about his frightened parents in their

6

neat flat, blameless. How the hell did it end up as bad as this?

Anyway.

Even later. Dog-tired. But not bored. Not on this shift.

Seventy-three minutes and twenty-three seconds to go.

The last 999 call is in a dull little town acting as a dormitory for the big international airport nearby. Not much happens here. Supposedly.

We're off out to a female – fifties – fainted in an art gallery. An *art* gallery? GP on scene – reports pulse very weak and irregular. Patient in and out of consciousness. The weak and irregular pulse in a woman that young is serious – could be a heart attack. We set off. Can't help wondering why an art gallery's open now and what a GP's doing there.

On scene we're led through the gallery, which is a large room with – not surprisingly – lots of pictures on the walls. There are at least fifty people in the room – all ages – the men wearing sharp suits and the women made up and wearing very low-cut dresses. Everyone's standing around the edges of the room, holding drinks and looking rather embarrassed, saying nothing.

Looks like a racy cocktail party gone wrong.

In the middle of the room – with no one anywhere near it – is something that looks like a tan leather gymnasium pommel horse with lots of belts, buckles and straps attached to it.

What *is* this place?

7

We're led to the patient, who's been moved to a side room. As we enter, the woman who turns out to be the GP – also in a low-cut dress – rushes past us and out of the door without saying a word.

It's not a heart attack, thank goodness. Davina's a nice lady, polite, with short blonde hair. She's wearing a black T-shirt, a black leather skirt and enormous black boots. She's making a good recovery – pulse is coming back strong. There's been no chest pain or shortness of breath. Her ECG, the electronic picture of the heart that we can look at, looks good.

As we assess her we see that her back and shoulders are covered with hundreds of tiny scratches and welts, as if she's been dragged through a rose bush ten times.

Val shoots me a look. *What the fuck is going on here?*

The patient's up for the night with a friend – another buxom lady in another low-cut dress.

—Has this ever happened before? Have you fainted before?

—Yes, when I've been running or exercising hard.

—But you've not been exercising hard tonight?

—Well… no.

She starts to look embarrassed and the penny finally drops.

This is an S&M club. Sadomasochism. Is that right? (Not even sure how to spell it.) Our patient is the 'victim' (presumably willingly), tied to the pommel horse somehow and thrashed to buggery with God knows what while everyone else looks on sipping their drinks politely. Nice. Not my cup of tea and very strange, but we're far too polite to comment. Takes all sorts. Didn't realise women did this sort of thing. Didn't really realise men did it, for that matter.

I try to phrase things delicately.

—Would it be fair to say your pulse might have been a little elevated by what was going on tonight?

—Well yes. Maybe we were going at it a bit strong.

—Maybe go at it a bit less strong next time?

(You should always give patients advice on how to manage their condition.)

—Yes, I think I will. Maybe give it up altogether.

Off we go.

The hospital – like a lot of them – appears to have been designed by a child with attention deficit disorder, the architect having an epileptic fit. Departments, corridors, lifts and wards all over the place, in no order at all. To get from one side to the other you have to take two different lifts, and cross a street. You could lose an army in here.

We take the patient to A&E, and hand her over to Fatima, one of the regular triage nurses. Triage nurses are usually the first hospital person the patient sees. Most are warm and welcoming and lovely. Fatima's... a bit different. She looks a little like Oddjob from *Goldfinger*. A large lady, ever so slightly menacing, she manages to look expressionless and disapproving at the same time – both of us and of the patients. (I'm sure she's lovely really.) I explain the faint, the irregular pulse, and as delicately as I can, the S&M thrashing. It's a bit like being a lawyer, in court defending a client before a judge. Fatima just stares, then writes *unwell patient* on the triage form.

All human life, as I said.

On the way out a colleague shouts cheerfully:

—Don't use the coffee machine! One of the NFAs (no fixed abode) was taking the spoons out earlier, licking them and putting them back!

Nice. (Makes a change from drinking the alcohol gel I suppose.)

End of shift and good night.

When the going gets tough – we're out of here.

We go back to the station – a huge, cavernous building with two sets of double doors that you drive in and out of. Ambulances come in one end and out the other, like sausages. Old and a bit dirty. Occasionally a pigeon flies in and we have to shoo it out. The station tells you a bit about the service. There are pictures on the walls of ambulances parked in formation, back in the 1970s and 80s and 90s. In the days when ambulance crews washed the ambulances, kitted them out, cleaned the station, even sat down and had a meal together. Nowadays, we're so busy that teams of people do all that for us – we collect our ambulances at the start of the shift and we're off out and might not see the station again until twelve or thirteen hours later. Though sometimes, on quieter nights, you can open up little cupboard rooms around the station and find old abandoned equipment and stuff in them, decades old. There's probably a body in there somewhere. Or someone living there. Maybe a patient?

I tell one of the bosses about the shift.

He's a very tall, thin man, slightly frightening and balding, called Len. Ex-forces, in the job a million years. A man of staring eyes and whispered words, unsmiling. Whatever bit of the forces he was in may not have been the Charm School Corps. He's retired now. Modern ambulance officers are a little more… cuddly, I suppose. He ponders the jobs a few minutes, then gives his stock response to a lot of things.

—Stupid buggers.

—I felt sorry for them, says Val. Especially the one who's mentally ill.

Len stares at her.

—What d'you want to feel sorry for him for? He's a nutter.

I get home about midnight – dog-tired – as Jo's going to bed. The kids who I left too early to see this morning are long in bed and I won't see them tonight. I pour myself an industrial-sized whisky. There might be another after that.

Jo looks at me.

—You know you're drinking too much, don't you?

This is the life. Just another long, crazy shift. Ours not to reason why, ours just to bitch and moan and wonder how the hell we all ended up here. What's the Talking Heads song? 'Once in a Lifetime'?

And you may ask yourself:

How did I get here?

2

COMMUNICATION

I joined the ambulance service in 2003 because I thought it would give me the sort of job I wanted. Something where you can make a difference. I may have a low boredom threshold. The service is rarely boring.

Up to then I'd had not exactly what you'd call a successful career. I only got to university because my girlfriend dumped me and went off to university herself, so I thought I'd better do the same. But I still didn't have much of a clue, so I followed my parents into journalism. Which I wasn't very good at.

I started doing shifts on the diary column of a well-known paper. I was so terrified my first morning I had to drink vodka before I went in to work just so I didn't shake too much. I was supposed to write fun snippets of news about famous people, but I didn't know any. The first piece I wrote ended up libelling someone so badly she won undisclosed damages in the High Court. I was told 'undisclosed' means at least five figures.

I never went back.

I decided to play it safe and went to work on a boring magazine called *Fish Trader*, about people who trade in...

fish. The only interesting thing about working there was that along the corridor you had other magazines with titles like *Disaster Management*, which sounded fun.

From there I moved to Scotland, to work on a local paper, which was more like being a proper reporter, although I couldn't understand most of the accents. It's difficult to quote people when you haven't a clue what they said. Good training for talking to people in pain and distress now, though.

Then I found out my mother was dying of cancer, and that changed things.

I left to live with her back in England. She lived alone. I spent a year watching her die in front of my eyes. That was probably good training for the ambulance service too. Just before she died she said the last year of her life had been the best.

I managed to get shift work on national newspapers after that, but never really had the confidence. I could never think of ideas for news stories, and felt frightened of most of the other people in the office. All of them seemed to have gone to Oxford or Cambridge or both. Sometimes I had to take a pill just to go and talk to the news editor or pick up the phone. So I left and painted houses and moved furniture. I don't miss journalism.

Reporting and ambulance work, asking people questions and trying to make sense of what they tell you, do have similarities. In news reporting, you're going out to people, trying to understand what's happened to them, and telling the readers. With ambulance work, you've got to find out what's happened a bit more quickly, then do something about it.

Then report to the hospital. Otherwise it's much the same thing. Sometimes just talking to people is the most important thing.

Sometimes their lives depend on it...

Douglas

Monday morning.

I apologise to any cardiologists, doctors or paramedics reading, but I may have invented a medical procedure. Maybe.

Called to a male, sixties, chest pains.

The symptoms are classic. Crushing central chest pain, radiating into left arm and jaw. Short of breath and dizzy and pale. Needs to go to the loo, sense of doom. Textbook stuff. Douglas is a tall, quite slim gent, alone in the house and very calm and pleasant. But it looks like a heart attack, and he knows it.

After he's been to the loo, we give him oxygen and aspirin and a spray in the mouth that takes a little of the pain away, then pop him on the carry chair and wheel him out to the ambulance. Once we've wired him up to the monitor, there's little room left for doubt. His ECG has what's known in the trade as massive ST elevation – another classic sign. At the hospital they'll do blood tests, but basically, if it walks like a duck and talks like a duck…

The doctors can give drugs that break up the clot, or even stick a tube into his veins to suck the thing out, but at the moment it's close to killing him.

So off to the hospital we go with lights and sirens flashing. Val's driving.

On the way in I do my best to reassure him, which isn't difficult. He seems quite calm and sensible. I can't imagine that I would be, in his situation. The spray has taken away some of the pain and he can breathe better, and I think he's gone into crisis mode – he knows exactly what's going on, and is almost waiting to find out what's going to happen. (I suppose it's not much fun having a heart attack, but probably the last thing you'd call it is boring.)

Anyway, all the way in I monitor him on the ECG and keep him talking. The ST elevation is getting bigger and bigger and the heart rhythm is becoming faster and more irregular as the heart is being damaged and becoming distressed, but he's still with us. It's only a three-minute drive in, and we've phoned ahead so they know we're coming.

We arrive at the hospital and wheel him into the resus bay (where the really ill people go), where a doctor and nurse are waiting to receive him. They both settle down either side of him, trying to get a needle into one of his veins to draw off blood and to give drugs. One's concentrating on his left arm, the other on the right. His veins are proving difficult, so for several minutes neither of them is looking at or talking to him, and this is when a strange thing happens.

In order to explain I need to go into a bit of detail. Apologies for the ignorance of what follows. Normal healthy hearts – as I understand it – generally don't just stop. They don't usually go from beating happily one second to stopped the next, except in the very old. They usually, or at least often, go from a normal heart beat into one of two rhythms: ventricular tachycardia, or more commonly ventricular fibrillation. With the first the heart's going so fast no blood gets in, so none can get pumped round the body (so you die) and with the second the heart starts jerking away in an uncoordinated fashion. Same result. Either way you're dead.

17

Only once you're good and dead some time will the heart slow down and actually stop.

So often with people who've just 'died' there's a period where their heart is doing one of the two things above. This is why people are given electric shocks. The shock will stop the heart doing either of these things above, and hopefully it will settle back to a normal rhythm.

Hey presto.

You were dead, now you're alive.

But if you haven't got a machine handy for giving electric shocks, a big fat punch in the chest can also do the trick. It's called a precordial thump. The effect is the same.

What I have invented (I think) is the precordial conversation.

Back in the resus room, the doctor and nurse are still busy trying to get needles in the patient's arms, while I'm watching the monitor. The patient's awake, but then goes even greyer and his head slumps to one side and his eyes close. I can see on the monitor that his heart rhythm is breaking up into ventricular fibrillation. This is the point at which he's technically dying, I suppose.

So I shout at him. Very loudly.

Something like what's your wife's name? He appears to wake up, shakes his head slightly, and tells me the answer. The rhythm on the monitor settles back down again.

Then a minute later, the same thing happens. He goes grey, his head slumps to one side, and the rhythm on the monitor breaks up. Dead again.

I shout at him again. Are you comfortable? Or something.

He shakes his head, wakes up, and the rhythm settles down.

Val's cleaning the stretcher. She can't see his face or the monitor. She gives me one of her looks. *What the fuck is wrong with you?*

I wonder how long we can go on like this.

—*What's your favourite colour?*

—*Who's going to win the FA Cup?*

—*Do you like ice cream?*

The answer's probably not long, but it definitely seems to work a couple of times before the doctors and nurses finish what they're doing and they can start shouting at him and keeping him busy and not dying. So we say goodbye and wish him luck and walk out of resus and into medical history, having invented the precordial conversation.

Like I said. Maybe.

Part of the reason I failed in journalism was I was terrible at job interviews. At one I saw the news editor of a major Sunday paper on a hot August day. I began to sweat so heavily rivers were running down my face. The editor looked concerned, as if I might have malaria, and asked if I was all right. Another time I went for a job with a big charity. My research was going to the library to look them up and find out they were the largest pressure group in the UK. One of the panel was an enormously fat woman.

—What do you know about us?

—I know you're a pressure group.

—What else?

—You're large, I said. Very large.

Silence.

Shit.

Even with a bit of experience, in this job, it's very easy to say the wrong thing. It's called foot-in-mouth disease. Val's often very helpful in pointing it out to me.

Val

When I joined the service there was a strict progression of experience before they let you loose on an emergency ambulance. (There still is.) First you did patient-transport work, ferrying people in and out of hospital for booked appointments. Then if you wanted to move to A&E you had to do a two-month course to become a trainee ambulance technician. You worked as a TAT for a year, always with someone more experienced. Then you had a two-day assessment to see what you were like, hopefully followed by qualification. After that you were let loose – allowed to work with someone who was less experienced than you.

You are *in charge*.

The first day of doing this – I'd been in the service about three years – was frightening. My first day in charge was a while ago now, with a trainee – Valerie. We had dead bodies both ends of the shift, my blood pressure went through the roof, but I think we got away with it.

Val's a bit like me, falling into the service after various jobs – airline stewardess, office worker – hating them all. I think she worked in a zoo once, which she quite liked. I bet that was good training for the job.

Val and I stayed together after this, as regular crewmates, for a while. You learn to depend on each other. You end up knowing the other's opinion on everything from Islamic fundamentalism to emulsion paint. Having a good solid crewmate's like having a good left leg. It's difficult without it.

Monica and Gordon

Midnight.

We're called to a female, twenties, in labour, childbirth imminent. This is not an unusual type of call, but the next bit is. They're in a field.

Or rather, parked beside one.

—Shit, says Val.

What's happened is she's gone into labour, so they've made a break for the hospital, but then the baby's decided not to play ball. It's playing I'm coming out now! The trouble is they don't know where they are or what road they're on, and so they've got right royally lost.

So we have an interesting ten minutes or so driving on blue lights up and down the road, looking for them. We come off the motorway. We go back on. No sign of them. At this rate the bloody thing will be collecting its old age pension before we find them.

Eventually, from up on the motorway, we see the van in the moonlight, hazards on, out in the country in the middle of nowhere. Five minutes later we pull up behind. Inside the scene is… novel. Mum is a young girl, naked from the waist down. She's already given birth while driving along, and the poor sausage has fallen out and landed in a heap in the footwell of the van before they even had time to stop. There's what looks like a massive Irish Wolfhound, or maybe a small horse, going bonkers in the back.

—Woof!

22

The whole inside is filthy. It's obviously a well-used vehicle, an old camper van, and hasn't been cleaned or tidied in years. Mud everywhere. Baby's now wrapped up in an old towel which doesn't look too clean either and is being cuddled by Mum.

The problem is the placenta hasn't been delivered yet, and we need to get Mum out and on to the ambulance, and the baby properly wrapped up in something that doesn't look like it's used to dry off the beast in the back. Luckily the police have arrived behind us, so they close off the road, so that we can draw alongside, and they hold up a blanket while we get the stretcher out and get Mum and baby on board. Not that there's anyone around here, anyway.

I go round to tell the person sitting in the van with her what we're going to do. He's an old man, maybe sixty or seventy, and looks Middle-eastern. Balding but with a pony tail. Maybe he's her father? He can hardly hear me over the dog.

—Woof!

—Are you a relative?

—I'm the father.

—*Her* father?

—No, the baby's father.

—Woof!

Shit.

Brilliant. Val mouths at me. *Fantastic. Well done.*

I've put my foot in it. Not for the first time. Oh well. Never mind.

As we get her on board and he follows us into the hospital, it's the elephant in the room – or ambulance – all the way in. We try and give the midwives a bit of a discreet warning so they don't blow their own feet off like I did, but it's difficult. Funny old world.

Funny *very* old world.

Mum and baby are doing fine when Dad arrives, thankfully dogless, shuffling in looking confused, every inch the mad professor. The midwives make everyone comfortable and test the newborn to make sure it hasn't suffered from the unscheduled rolling around on the filthy floor.

My crewmate and I wish them all well and leave, wondering how soon we'll be back out to him with dementia or something.

The interview with my boss Len for the ambulance service was pretty successful, compared with the charity fiasco. For some reason I didn't feel so nervous. Maybe I knew I wanted the job. Or that I might be OK at it.

Did I mind blood, vomit, faeces? Was I hard-working? Did I like people?

No, no, no, yes, yes.

Was I reliable and good in a crisis?

Yes and maybe.

Did I have any unsightly or offensive tattoos?

I looked at his arms, covered in tattoos from elbow to wrist.

No, but I can get some if you want.

It was pretty much the only time I had ever seen him laugh.

Silly bastard.

I was in.

* * *

So that's how I started.

The service itself started earlier. Wikipedia will tell you the first recorded ambulance was a hammock-based cart affair ferrying around leprosy and psychiatric patients a thousand years ago. Presumably everyone else had to walk. The first emergency ambulances were used by the Spanish 500 or so years later, and London had a civilian service for cholera patients a few hundred years after that. All pulled by horses or people. Then late in the nineteenth century came the first motor ambulances, before Ernest Hemingway hit the PR button with *A Farewell to Arms*.

Only in the 1950s, though, did the emphasis shift from regarding ambulances as means of transporting patients to mobile hospitals for treating them. Since then the pace has hotted up. Equipment and procedures change almost by the year, reflecting changes in medical thinking.

But one thing never changes. There's always a form to fill out. Paperwork.

There are forms for every patient. If they don't go to hospital, another one. If they're septic, another. If they've died, another. I have a joke if patients are not sure they want to go to hospital.

—Let's do the paperwork; then we'll both have died of old age.

And there's an endless variety of jobs. An endless variety of things that can go wrong in this life.

Where else could you take two people into the hospital on the same shift? One who's suffered a cardiac arrest while driving and crashed into a building. We got him back. (Good job, said Len.) The other who's fainted, frightened he was allergic to his cheese and onion sandwich.

(For fuck's sake, said Len.)

One of the reasons I like the Health Service is I always wanted to be a comedian. This isn't as strange as it sounds. My oldest friend used to run comedy clubs all over the place, and I used to help out on the door taking money. This was back in the nineties. A lot of people who would become household names performed. I used to yearn to have the bottle to get up on the stage and make people laugh, but I never did. In the ambulance service you can step on and off the stage whenever you like. You can be funny when you need to be, and serious when you don't. A lot of times when people phone 999, they want someone to come along and take charge of a bad situation, not panic, and make it better. An amazing number of times, a joke succeeds in all three.

—Haven't I seen your face before?

—Yes, on *Crimewatch*.

Or:

—You're a smooth driver.

—I'm even better when I've sobered up.

Or:

—I was in hospital last week with me legs.

—Better than being in there without them.

That sort of thing. You sort of have to be there, but they do work. And obviously we've got bandages and drugs and oxygen and stuff for when a joke isn't quite enough. One of the things you learn is when to make the joke and when not to. Sometimes Val gives me a look.

It's time you shut up now.

You can't make a joke out of everything.

And it has to be said, sometimes it's the patients who say the funniest things.

Kenny

Another shift with Val.

We're called to a man, fifties, outside his flat in town. He's a known self-harmer and he's cut his neck.

So far, doesn't sound too exciting. We go out to a lot of self-harmers and they don't usually do too much damage. Usually just cuts and scratches deep enough to show a little blood and let the pain out, as one of them once told me.

But this guy's a little different. When we get there there's a very worried-looking copper holding a dressing to the man's neck. The patient is sitting on the pavement with his back against the wall. His face is white in the darkness and he's wearing a dark red tracksuit.

Only it's not a dark red tracksuit. It's a white tracksuit, absolutely covered in blood. Soaked. He's sitting in a pool of it.

Blimey, we think, and switch into hurry-up mode.

The patient's still conscious and breathing, and he hasn't actually cut his own throat, so he's still able to breathe. But he's very close to fainting because his blood pressure's collapsed due to the fact he's sitting in most of it. We get him on some oxygen and onto a stretcher with his feet raised so what little blood's left goes to his head where it's needed. A paramedic who's backing us up gets a line and some fluids in him with difficulty and we relieve the poor copper, also looking rather pale, and get a new dressing on his neck. Then it's off to hospital.

—What the bloody hell happened?

Kenny has a history of depression, alcohol dependence and self-harm, and often cuts his arms or neck with a Stanley knife, but like most people just makes small cuts. Tonight he was (sort of) happily cutting away at the side of his neck when he realised things had gone too far and the blood's pissing out like a tap. He staggers out into the street and calls 999. A bit of a shock really, but maybe the brush with death will do him some good. Shake something up in his head.

I can't help thinking despite the self-harm, alcoholism and depression, he's still something of an optimist. He's unemployed, wearing a filthy old tracksuit drenched in blood, and he's got a drink problem. Val's in the back with him. She's young and beautiful and professional, and he doesn't know about the bad language.

—You going out with anyone? he asks on the way into hospital with the blue lights flashing.

—No, not at the moment.

—Would you go out with me?

—Well, let's get you to the hospital and sorted out first, shall we? Then we'll see.

At hospital Fatima manages to look expressionless and mystified at the same time. I think she often finds us – patients and ambulance staff – strange.

—He cut his *own* throat?

—Yes.

Unwell patient.

3

FREQUENT FLYERS

Friday evening – years ago. I'm petrified, as frightened as I've ever been in my life. I joined the ambulance service eighteen months ago, and now it's my first-ever shift on a proper, front-line, A&E, emergency ambulance. Tonight, real people – the poor sods – will depend on me to look after them; their lives will be in my hands. I can't quite believe it – why did I ever sign up to this?

Fuck!

Anyway, I'm crewed up with a nice experienced woman, Denise, who no doubt will look after me, but it's still terrifying. I've opted to attend for the first six hours of the shift – best to get it over with – so I'll be in the back with the patients. Oh my God. We sign on and the shift starts at 7 o'clock, and after that we're just waiting for the first job.

I'm shitting myself.

Nothing happens for the first half an hour, and this even makes it worse. Denise sits watching *EastEnders* or something, perfectly calm, she's seen it all before. I sit watching the screen but taking nothing in, trying to stop my heart hammering away. And then it happens. Our pagers go off and we have a job. I jump up and get in the ambulance, wondering if I'll have a heart attack or throw up first.

Billy

Halfway to the scene the details of the job come over. Male, forties, blood gushing from ear. Conscious and breathing.

Jesus Christ, I think, what's this? 'Blood gushing from his ear'? What from? An injury? Assault? A cerebral bleed? Bloody hell. What on earth do I do?

Denise remains icily calm and says nothing as the blue lights flash and she drives to the job, which has been called in from a phone box in the town centre. Then we see the call box with the caller still in it. All she does is sigh quietly.

—It's Billy Watts.

Billy Watts? *Billywatts?* What does that mean? A person? An illness? A condition?

I jump out and head towards the patient. He's rough-looking, in his forties, dressed in dirty clothes, with a tiny trickle of dried blood coming from his ear – nothing else. Drunk and filthy.

I lead him to the ambulance and get him on board and wash his ear, which has a tiny scratch on it, with shaking hands and take his pulse. He doesn't seem unwell otherwise but is obviously drunk. My crewmate looks on silently, her face a mask.

—Shall we head off? she says.

If we don't take him to hospital now, he'll phone back later with 'chest pains' or 'suicidal thoughts' or something. He likes going to the hospital, and he'll keep phoning back till we take him. Might as well get it over with. This is the way it works with some people, though I don't know this yet.

33

So off we go to hospital. Fatima stares at me.

—Why you bring him here? Nothing wrong with him.

It turns out he's a regular visitor to the hospital, usually drunk, complaining of self-inflicted injuries or no injuries at all. But I've got him to hospital alive, and therefore done my job, and survived myself, and so we're up and running.

I even took his blood pressure on the way in to hospital.

—You did what? Denise asks.

—I took his blood pressure.

—You bloody idiot. It's Billy Watts. You might've got your stuff dirty.

That was my first A&E job. Hardly exciting.

It was still useful, though. It taught me to expect the unexpected – there's a lot of unexpected in this job. And you learn there are a terrifying number of Billy Wattses in the world. People with little or nothing and blowing whatever they have.

People watch *Holby City* or *Casualty* and think every job is life-threatening and involves a plane crashing on to a train which ploughs into an orphanage, all on Christmas Eve. And you're trying to do the job thinking about splitting up with your partner or having a sex change or whatever. It isn't always like that. If it was you'd end up in a lunatic asylum. Or like Billy Watts.

In the airline trade you get people who are called 'frequent flyers', successful business people racking up the air miles attending conferences and going to meetings and whatnot. Successful, respectable, nice.

In the service we have frequent flyers too. But they are not always so nice. And they don't smell quite so good. People who call 999 for the wrong reasons, or no reasons, sometimes hundreds of times.

Some are in a desperate state. Some aren't.

Probably the most astonishing fact about the service is the degree to which it's abused by them. Some have worked out that if certain buzz phrases are used – 'chest pains' or 'short of breath' – the service gets all Pavlovian and sends an ambulance to check them out, no matter what. Even if they've called hundreds of times before, this might be the one time they're genuine. Each area has what is called its 'regulars' (like a pub) who sometimes call every day. I heard one elderly lady in our area had had a total of something like £400,000 worth of ambulance visits over a few years. At anything up to £400 a call-out, that means she's called an ambulance over a thousand times. And we still go to her.

Another thing you learn is that ambulance crews have a slightly ambivalent attitude to them. Yes they make us angry. But we also talk about them a lot in the crew room, swapping horror stories, like exasperated parents.

Almost as if we're fond of them.

They may be bastards, as Len might say, but they're OUR bastards.

Dave

The king of the frequent flyers in the area where I used to work was Dave.

Usually violent, abusive and drunk, Dave was a legend, the top of the charts, the big cheese. He was the Elvis of the frequent flyers. And a right royal pain in the arse.

Friday afternoon.

Called to a male, forties, chest pains.

He's living in a filthy unkempt flat in the poorer area of town, with an enormous dog in the kitchen, who luckily appears quite friendly. We say hello. Dave's lying on the sofa, drunk but reasonably coherent, surrounded by empty bottles and full ashtrays. The bottles are huge blue cider bottles. I look at the nearest one. It says 'Sharing Bottle' on it. Do me a favour.

—I've got chest pains. I need to go to hospital.

—Oh really.

Over the course of the next ten minutes we ascertain Dave's chest pains (if they exist at all) are provoked by a cough and certainly not cardiac. They're more likely to be related to the million cigarettes he smokes every day. None of his other observations point to anything cardiac. We advise him to see his doctor and leave.

Five minutes later we're called back to the same address. Male, forties, chest pains. Back we go. Again we wire him up to the ECG but it still shows nothing – just a normal heartbeat. Again we advise a visit to the GP and leave.

I notice a packet of Diazepam on the sofa amongst all the fags and bottles.

—You know, Dave, if you keep mixing those with booze, one day you're going to fall asleep on that sofa and just stop breathing.

Five minutes up the road the call comes pinging through. Male, forties, not breathing.

I stare at the screen.

—I just told him that! I just told him! And if he's not breathing how come he's managed to phone a sodding ambulance?

—Bastard! screams Val.

Back we go.

Same old story. He's still claiming chest pains and wants to go to hospital. It's obvious there's nothing the hospital could do for him. All he would do is sit there, swearing at the nurses. He's done it a hundred times before. Once again we leave, and once again, five minutes up the road he calls again. Male, forties, short of breath. This is the fourth call.

Back we go. As before there's nothing wrong with him that a bath and a bullet in the head wouldn't cure. But he keeps calling, and we keep sending. While Val diverts his attention I pick up the phone he uses to call us. I take it through to the kitchen and offer it to the dog, hoping he'll chew it up. The dog isn't interested. I can't really stamp on it, so I take it back through to the front room and slip it down the side of the sofa cushion so it's not in view. Then, finally, we say goodbye and get out of there.

He doesn't call back.

Micky

People can get that *Holby City* or *Casualty* impression of the job. But sometimes you do get a job that sounds like it's straight off the telly.

It's near the end of an unremarkable shift on the car and then something comes over the computer which makes me prick up my ears.

Female, thirties, on ground and covered in blood, CPR being performed. CPR? This doesn't sound good. There's lots of other stuff as well. Patient lying on grass outside house, caller distressed, screaming.

Jobs like this you go like fuck. Drive it like you stole it.

Which is what I proceed to do. The job's eight miles north and I nearly kill at least one person on the way there. The Critical Care Paramedic is coming up from ten miles south and he probably nearly kills two. The patient's down a windy road through a housing estate, and I scream down it red-lining the engine and stamp on the brakes and turn the corner to find…

…nothing. Zilch.

The square root of fuck all.

It's a hoax. There's a paramedic truck already there and a police car and not much else. The caller's a local nutter who does it all the time – the police recognise the number. They'll be going round his house in a minute to have a little word. Apparently he's so loopy there's not much point in trying to prosecute him, he'd probably start barking at the judge or licking the floor or crapping in the dock or something.

We all stand down as the CCP turns up, smoke coming out of his wheel arches and his ears. Not happy.

I'm just glad the call's got me off on time. My car stinks of burnt clutch for days afterwards.

We go out to all sorts of unfortunate people, but in a way the ones I tend to feel for aren't those that have died of a heart attack, or smashed themselves up in a car crash. I sometimes feel sorriest for people like Billy, Micky and Dave. It's not how you die that's important. It's how you live.

4

EMERGENCY ADMISSIONS

One of the problems, or tragedies, about the modern NHS is that the wartime generation, that defeated Hitler, never complained and never called an ambulance because they didn't want to make a fuss, is dying out. To be replaced by today's me-generation – products of the Welfare State from cradle to grave, who call an ambulance at the drop of a hat because they've scratched their finger opening their dole cheque. (A bit of an exaggeration but you get the picture.)

This can occasionally catch you out. There are still patients who should be much *more* frequent flyers...

Bob and Mildred

Evening.

We're down in a dormitory town which is, to be frank, a bit of a dump, with more than its fair share of welfare scroungers, druggies and alkies. We get a call to a male – no age given. Has picked a spot and it's still bleeding.

—Oh for fuck's sake, says Val. 'Picked a spot and it's still bleeding'? You're having a laugh, aren't you?

I shake my head and we drive off to the job in the ambulance and a cloud of disgust.

I don't spot the early warning signs. The house is in one of the town's 'respectable' enclaves, neat and well cared for, and when I knock the door is answered by an elderly lady, white hair, just like your lovely grandma.

—Hello dear.

—Hello, my love. What's the problem?

—Oh he's in the back, through there. Thanks for coming. Sorry to get you out. He's picked a spot and there's a bit of blood.

—OK my love, let's have a look at him.

I go through to the back room, still slightly peeved but determined not to show it, but that feeling doesn't last long.

The back room is a bloodbath, claret all over the floor, sprayed up the walls in places, all over a chair. The claret's previous owner (or container) is an elderly gent, Bob, presumably the lady's husband, lying flat on his back, white as a sheet.

Bloody hell.

42

He's still conscious, though only just, and when I even try to sit him up, let alone stand him up, he faints dead away. I lie him back down on the floor, put an oxygen mask on him, and put his feet up on a chair, to get what little blood's left in him up to his heart and brain.

He hasn't picked a spot. He's nicked an artery in his leg, and because it's an artery the blood has pissed out all over the place. There must be literally pints of it all over the floor, and he's in shock – basically there isn't enough blood left in his body for his heart to pump it up to his brain and keep him conscious if he sits or stands up.

It's serious but manageable, with the right treatment. Without it, he could die. I get a dressing on the wound, though it's not bleeding much any more, and call for backup. He needs a paramedic to put a line in so we can get fluids into him, and he needs to go off to hospital lying flat, so the leg can be fixed.

He'll probably need a blood transfusion as well, he's lost so much.

We get him packaged up and off to hospital, and I stay behind to try and clear up a bit of the mess on the floor, and call someone to come and be with the wife so she's not left alone terrified. True to form, she doesn't seem that worried anyway.

—Sorry to call you out again, darling. Would you like a cup of tea?

I tell her to sit down. I'll make the tea.

Enid

After qualifying, the next stage in your progress in ambulance life is working on your own, in a fast-response car. You're supposed to get to the job first and assess it and stabilise it.

You're 'it'.

And I'm doing it for the first time tonight. No Val to hold my hand. Or anyone else.

This is hard-core stuff. You make the decisions. You have nobody to fall back on, nobody to help. At least without calling up on the radio. Some people in the job decades longer than me still don't like doing the car.

I'm shitting myself. I go over the thing with a fine-tooth comb, making sure all the equipment is there. There's lots of it, the car's groaning with it – looks like I'm off on holiday. Only I'm not.

Luckily, the dispatcher is a friend of mine, so I call him and tell him it's my first night, and he promises to be gentle with me. And he is, bless him.

First job of the night is an elderly lady in a restaurant, cut leg.

Not too frightening. She's a lovely old dear, being taken out for an evening meal by her family in the pub. And she's hungry.

In the restaurant she's sitting at the table, studying the menu. She's nicked a varicose vein in her leg and the blood's pouring out over her foot and the floor, while her family look concerned. I bandage the wound up with a pressure dressing. She needs to go to the hospital but she doesn't want to go.

—I've been waiting for this for ages. I'm hungry. I'm not going to hospital.

—Please Mum, your leg's bleeding. You need to go.

—No I don't. I need a prawn cocktail and a main course. And pudding. What's everyone else having?

It takes an age for them to persuade her to go.

Elliot

Midnight.

It's been the usual horrendous Saturday night.

Mainly following the police around from job to job. Drunks fighting, so they've got minor facials and the police want them 'checked out' in the hope we'll take them off their hands and down the hospital. Or drunks unconscious, in which case the police refuse to have them in their cells and *insist* we take them down the hospital. The ambulance service gets on a lot better with the police than with the fire brigade – the police are as busy as us. But sometimes the relationship's a bit like an old married couple.

Anyway, around midnight, we get called to the multi-storey car park in the middle of the town's shopping complex, to an elderly male, jumped off the roof.

Elliot.

We're only at the hospital, two minutes up the road.

An elderly black gent, speechless and wearing a high-visibility jacket – some sort of security guard – meets us and leads us around the corner and onto a piece of bushy grass next to the building. I glance up at the car-park wall beside me. It's at least four storeys high. Maybe 60 feet.

Shit.

The patient is lying on the grass on his back, unconscious but still breathing, legs twisted under him. We get a collar on him and some oxygen, and the paramedic gets an IV line into him. This sort of impact will almost certainly have caused massive, probably fatal, internal bleeding. Me and my crewmate are getting the truck as near as we can and unloading the equipment we'll need to get him on to the stretcher.

The patient is an elderly man, dressed in pyjamas, dressing gown and slippers. What the hell is he doing here? The poor security guy still staring at the scene horrified is in shock. He holds out a half-empty black bottle. It's morphine sulphate, a powerful painkiller of the type given to patients with things like terminal cancer.

—I found this on the roof.

The poor sod. It turns out he was sitting in his office on the ground floor when he saw the old man come into the car park and go to the staircase. He wondered what he was doing here – maybe he was lost or confused. So he followed him up the stairs, looking in on each floor to see where he'd gone. Eventually he got to the roof and found him there on the edge. When he approached to see if he could help, the man jumped.

There are no private houses immediately around here. So he's either walked a while to get here, or perhaps got out of the hospital up the road. Maybe the morphine is because he's got a terminal illness, and just wants a quick way out.

In which case, sadly, he may well get it. He's still breathing on the ambulance, but when we push on his pelvis, there's a grating feeling. This is called crepitus, and it's the feeling of broken bone ends crunching together – his pelvis is smashed, and at his age he's unlikely to survive that, never mind what's gone on inside.

But he's still with us, so we leave the poor security guard for the police to take care of and we scream off up to the hospital.

Once there we hand over to the staff in the resus bay to do what they can for him, then go and get a cup of tea and try to forget him. Which takes some doing.

5

FEAR

I joined the service in 2003, but maybe the training started earlier than that.

I was born in London in 1965.

My parents were what was called at the time 'interesting' but would now be called 'dysfunctional'. Or nuts. My mother was a freelance writer, married to another writer. He wasn't my father. My father was yet another writer, deputy editor of a national newspaper. He already had a wife, and two children. And a dog. So I ended up in a family that included half-brothers, half-sisters and maybe even half-dogs.

Complicated. It was a mess. Like living in a lunatic asylum sometimes.

When I was a boy, me and my mum lived in a dirty ramshackle flat in south London with a Jack Russell terrier, a boiler that blew up all the time and a series of demented cats. Also a sea of empty wine bottles. All of these things were more or less connected.

My father was a funny and witty and kind man, but spent a lot of his time with his head in the clouds, thinking about politics and economics and that sort of thing. Also a heavy drinker. I think he probably first thought of his relationship with my mother as an affair – nothing too serious. But she had other ideas, and then his children, so it didn't work out like that. My father never left his wife, which meant we only saw him every other weekend after my stepfather left, weekends which often descended into a drunken fight between him and my mother about when (if ever) he was going to leave his wife and come live with his second-class family. (My mother's words, not mine.) He never did, and I used to dread the sound of his motorbike turning up outside the house, knowing the peace was about to be shattered.

My stepfather left when I was about five. When she wasn't having rows with my father, my mother managed a few with him as well, though he was quieter. Both men got on fine.

The whole messy stew was pickled in alcohol. My parents would be described nowadays as problem drinkers, though they usually never had much of a problem with it. They were fun, don't get me wrong. They worked, and there was a lot of laughter and affection when they weren't smashing bottles over each other's heads or throwing food around.

Freud said the ability to love and to work was a good guide to mental health. But I'd have liked a bit more than that.

And I ended up in the emergency ambulance service, which is a bit of a contrast. Life on an ambulance seems calm and ordered in comparison. Logical, sensible, rational.

Sometimes…

Fear

People always say you must see some things, doing your job. The nasty jobs with all the drama. They're sometimes right. People ask about them and want you to remember them, but the nasty ones are the ones you'd rather forget.

Darren

Dusk falling. Midwinter.

We're standing outside the ambulance station smoking. Me, my crewmate and Vicki, who's on the fast-response car, and isn't a flappable person. Her buzzer goes off to signal she has a job, so she goes and gets in her car to start the engine and look at the computer screen to see what it is.

Then she screams at me.

—Shit! Follow me!

—Eh? You what?

—Follow me! Follow me!

We follow her. The job comes over the computer within a minute. Man hanging in the woods. Next to the cemetery, just to make it even more ghoulish, as dusk falls. This is obviously on the time-critical side, so off we go.

We get there a bit behind Vicki. We can only see her lights, as she's driven to the very far side of the graveyard, near the woods, where the man who found the patient has led her. I sprint across the grass to meet her.

When we get to the patient, there's nothing to be done. Darren's a young man, only in his twenties or thirties, kneeling under a tree. A rope round his neck leads up to a branch about six feet up. There's an empty bottle of vodka on the ground at his feet, lots of cigarette butts. Maybe Dutch courage. There's nothing we can do. He's cold to the touch, and it's obvious he's been dead some time. Kneeling beside him doing the stupid paperwork, I can't help thinking about the finality of what he's done. We go out to a lot of overdoses where the patient's taken pills and called 999 because they want help. But there's no going back from a hanging. You can rebuild a lot of burnt bridges in this life. But not this fucking one.

By this time it's almost dark and the police have arrived. From our point of view there's little to be done. We need to take an ECG of his heart, just to show legally there's no activity and he's dead, then we can leave it to the police. They'll organise the undertakers to come and collect the body and inform the family. But there's still a few surprises in store.

First a woman comes suddenly through the woods, with a dog, clearly upset.

—Where is he?

It turns out the patient lived just on the other side of the woods, and left a suicide note. This woman, a friend or relative, has read it and rushed over, too late. Vicki and I go back to the ambulance to collect the ECG machine, then make our way back towards the patient, still hanging in the woods. By now it's almost completely dark, so we head towards the lights of the police torches flashing in the darkness.

I walk straight into the body of a man, kneeling down, hanging from a tree, just like the first. His head bumps against my chest. My heart nearly stops.

Jesus Christ, what's this? Another one?

It turns out the police have moved away from the body to examine a bench in the woods, surrounded by cigarette butts and another vodka bottle, where the unfortunate patient must have spent his last hour or so. The body I've bumped into is the original one, thank God.

The three of us do the stuff we've got to do, then get out of there as fast as we can.

There's an old Russian proverb:

*We are born in a meadow,
but we die in a dark wood.*

Bad things happen in woods.
(And not just to Russians.)

Ivan

Called to a male, thirties, fallen over with a head injury.

This turns out to be about as frightened as I've ever been doing this job. The location is a bugger for a start. The man's on a path deep in woods south of town. This is quite a large area of thick woodland with different paths running across it. In the end it turns out the nearest we can get is a deserted industrial estate where we park the ambulance and walk up a path through the woods for about a mile.

Eventually we come across the patient and a rather brave woman out walking her dog who's come across him. He's in his thirties, thin, naked from the waist up, and intoxicated of course. He's shaven-headed and has a large cut on his head where he fell on the pathway. He's really whipcord-thin, with staring eyes and loads of old scars on his head and arms. He may have been knocked out – she's not sure.

Nor is he, because he doesn't speak much English – he's Lithuanian. We explain that because of his head injury we'd like to take him to hospital for observation, and he seems quite happy with that. But first he has to get some belongings.

—Where from?

—You come. I show you.

So the three of us tramp through the woods off the path for a good few hundred yards in deep bracken.

Eventually we come across his 'home' just as it's starting to get dark. Maybe I'm just tired or something, but I start to feel uneasy. This isn't a home – it's a lair. A tiny clearing in

55

the woods, with two small tents opening on to it. Maybe one of the tents is for house guests, but there's no one there now. There's a clothes line between two trees, empty food packets, pill packets, and bottles all over the place. And it's freezing and getting dark. I look in one of the tents and see what looks like a huge hunting knife in a corner, while our friend pulls on a jumper, singing to himself and dancing all over the place.

It turns out he's been living here for over a year, all through last winter and well into this one. He used to have work on a farm, but not any more. God knows what he's living on. Tinned beans, pills and alcohol by the looks of it.

Val's a pretty tough cookie, but she's not the biggest person in the world, and the more I'm around Ivan, the more nervous I get. He's really nervy, twitchy and agitated, and spends half the time dropping into crouches and taking practice potshots at the woods. He says he used to be in the Lithuanian special forces (does Lithuania have special forces?) and shows me some sort of military ID card, so who knows? He says he got beaten up by the police there and 'had to get out'. He's been in England ever since, living rough.

Living rough deep in the woods and going stark staring bonkers, is what I think. I don't want to think about the damage he could do if he really lost it. I can imagine the paranoia taking over and him killing some poor sod out walking their dog in the woods one misty morning as he wakes up and thinks they're hunting him.

Anyway, maybe I'm just tired.

With a few more howls at the moon and a few more crouches and potshots at imaginary Russians, we manage to get him safely on the ambulance, and with me keeping a wary eye on him in the back, into hospital. And there we leave him in the waiting room, ticking away, eyes swivelling around, veins pumping in his head. I think I should report him to the police, but what for? He hasn't done anything wrong. Trouble is I can imagine him doing something very wrong. Very easily indeed.

But, at least, not while Fatima's around.

I wouldn't give him much of a chance against her.

Given my childhood, perhaps another reason I was drawn to this job is that it's simple. In any given situation there are protocols to follow. Learn the protocols and you're laughing.

This is rubbish, of course. One of the reasons to love the job is that despite all the protocols, all the training, all the times you've seen similar jobs before, something always turns up to surprise you.

Or frighten the bloody life out of you.

Like pretty much any other functioning organisation, the emergency ambulance service has a hierarchy, although to be fair things are fairly informal. And job titles change practically every week, in a deckchairs-on-the-*Titanic* sort of way. (I jest of course.) At the bottom (and most are better than me, certainly Val is) are Emergency Care Support Workers. Then Associate Practitioners. Next come Ambulance Technicians – my grade. Next up are Paramedics (which is what the public call anyone in a green uniform who doesn't work for Homebase anyway). Then you've got various grades of specialised Paramedic: Paramedic Practitioner, Critical Care Paramedic, Paramedic Who Does Magic and Speaks Urdu, that sort of thing.

Then you get the officers. The junior, the middle-ranking, and then you get to the exalted heights of the senior officers. From there you've got individual directors and board members, and above that the chief executive himself. The next grade up is God.

The other thing about the service is also universal. Senior officers are admired, respected, loved. (Obviously.) But you don't usually want people like them turning up on a job. It's a bit like your mother turning up to give advice while you're trying to lose your virginity.

Mrs C.

It's mid-morning and Val and I are driving through one of the local towns on our way to a cover point when a job comes through.

Female, fifties, collapsed in a car park near the hospital.

This is a dodgy call. The drunks aren't usually up and about and falling over this early, and especially not round here. Then the radio starts beeping. This is an even worse sign. It's usually the controller calling to say the job's turned into a resus – the patient's arrested. Uh oh.

—Romeo Two?

—Yes?

—Just to let you know, you're going out to Mrs C.

—Mrs C.?

—Yes. Mrs C.

—Fuck, says Val. Fuck, fuck, fuck.

Mrs C. is one of the A&E consultants in our area. She's nice and everything but she *is* a bit frightening. If brains were dynamite Val's and mine wouldn't even blow her eyelids open in the morning. She's probably forgotten more than we'll ever know. Lots of ambulance people don't even work in the town they live in, in case they go out to someone they know. We're going out to an expert in emergency medicine, in public, probably with something serious going on, maybe dead.

(No fucking pressure then.)

We scream round the corner to the car park, where we see a bunch of senior police officers and council people – the

59

people Mrs C. was meeting – all surrounding her lying on the floor. We screech to a stop, grab our equipment, and dive on her.

And luckily, thank the lord and the fates and all who are on high, she's all right. Fully conscious and already recovering from the faint – she's been unwell recently, which hasn't helped. She stares at us, doesn't say anything, and lets us get on with it.

In fact she's a model patient. We get her on the truck and do all the tests we can on her, then do most of them again, all a bit embarrassed. She just lies there with her eyes closed.

—Just do what you've got to do.

We take her into hospital, and make sure we don't have to queue up in the corridor before handing her over to Fatima, which earns us some brownie points. She smiles at me.

—Thanks, she says as we file out. Thanks a lot.

She shakes my hand.

High praise indeed.

6

ALCOHOL

My parents weren't the sort of people to become ambulance people. They weren't alcoholics; they were a bit more like drunks, sometimes. (Alcoholics go to meetings, as the T-shirt used to say.) They were writers, and most writers of their generation drank. You wrote and you drank. Not always in that order.

One night (when I was about seven years old) we were trying to persuade my mother to go to bed. It was about midnight, and she was drunk. A friend (another writer, also drunk) was trying to persuade her to come outside and carry on drinking with him. I'd managed to push him out of the flat and lock the door, and was trying to push my mother towards the bedroom. But the friend was outside on his knees, cooing through the catflap.

—I've got another bottle! Come out for a drink!

Eventually my mother appeared from the bedroom in a dressing gown, looking serious and sober.

—Right, this has gone on long enough. I'm going to go out there and tell him to go home.

The effect was only ruined by the fact she couldn't quite

stand up straight, and by the empty glass she was hiding behind her back.

Good training.

Growing up with people who drank and lived their lives as if they were in a lunatic asylum has given me some sympathy for patients, who often drink and are living their lives as if in a lunatic asylum too.

Charlie and Ellie

Friday morning.

First job of the shift is a 27-year-old female, abdominal pains and vomiting, alcohol withdrawal, malnourished.

Twenty-seven years old?

The patient is lying on the floor, retching uncontrollably, stick-thin. We get told some of the story. She's a long-term alcoholic (at twenty-seven!), hospitalised with the same symptoms last week. She's living in a hostel fifteen miles south, down in town 'visiting friends' but basically killing herself. All week since her last admission she's been drinking, eating nothing, and now for the last two days doubled up in agony and vomiting.

She's incontinent, with thick black, tarry faeces. This isn't normal digested food. It's blood. Her internal organs, liver and pancreas, are so inflamed they're causing her agony, and her stomach lining is bleeding. Her pulse is racing and her blood pressure's low – everything's collapsing. Her dyed blonde hair is matted with sweat and vomit and there are clusters of spots from a rash around her mouth. Apart from that, she's great.

We get the patient down on to the ambulance and settled and as comfortable as possible. From her I gather mum and stepdad live about 100 miles away, as does a big brother. She hasn't completely lost touch or fallen out with them, but 'doesn't want them to see her like this'.

—Do they know how bad things are?

—No, not really.

She refuses to give any details, never mind addresses or phone numbers, so there's no way to contact them anyway even if someone was allowed to. I think about this on the way in, while she sleeps awhile. What it really needs is a doctor to take over, phone her family, and for them to come and get her, take her to a clinic and commit her there, if necessary against her will, for months or even years, at enormous cost, where she can go through rehabilitation and get the nursing she's going to need. Then it will be years of therapy, psycho-analysis, call it what you will – again at vast expense – to iron out whatever's made her get this far. Even with all that there are no guarantees. And it's not going to happen.

Unfortunately it's pretty obvious what is.

When I go back into A&E later she's gone. Fatima says she's been sent home.

—She doesn't have a home – she lives in a hostel.

Fatima shrugs her shoulders. She was judged fit for discharge. That's it.

I never see her again.

I'm still thinking about her the following day when another one comes along.

The most common thing people ask about the ambu-lance service is how do you deal with the drunks and the alcoholics? The drunks are boring and annoying (but can be fun), but I have a lot of sympathy for the alcoholics. They're often not the same thing for a start. Alcoholics are often long past being happily drunk. That's probably a distant memory for them. They drink because they have to.

We're called to a male, thirty, who's had a fit.

The address is a bit of a dingy flat, where the patient lives with Mum. It's a sea of fag butts and empty cans. The cans are all over the floor and table, neatly stacked like an army. A brand of well-known lager – nothing else. I still remember the adverts when I was a kid. The amber nectar – like an angel crying on your tongue, Paul Hogan used to say.

Only she seems to be vomiting green bile over your face today.

He's dead white, shaking uncontrollably. He's had a fit for about five minutes, been vomiting continuously for days. He's due into a rehab clinic in a few weeks' time and the doctors have told him not to stop drinking until then. He's got to keep drinking the lager, his mum says almost cheerfully as she leads me to the front room. Like she's saying he's got to keep studying for his exams. Don't know if she knows how ill he is.

The trouble with booze or drugs is you get addicted to them, of course. So even if you want to get off them, you can't. Catch-22. My patient is in a Catch-33 situation. His central nervous system is dependent on alcohol, and without it he falls apart, shaking and shivering and having fits or convulsions. But the part of his body that's got to deal with it first – the liver and stomach and pancreas and whatnot – is fucked, had enough and is saying no more. Even though he needs the drink he can't get it, because he can't keep it down. Catch-33.

He needs to go into hospital, so they can manage the withdrawal with drugs that stop the fitting, and deal (if they can) with the internal bleeding that's going on somewhere in his wrecked stomach.

So it's off to hospital we go – the same hospital the 27-year-old female was discharged from only hours ago.

I wonder what'll happen to both of them.

I'm a pretty heavy drinker. Val's no stranger to a few sherbets. But we're teetotal compared to this lot.

7

ARGUMENTS

My mother was warm and funny, but often a heavy drinker and as disorganised in her own way as my father. She came from a large Catholic family from Birmingham or Bath, I never quite worked out which. She was a bit of a black sheep, leaving her family for London and a career in writing and journalism when she was barely out of her teens. She had a slightly artificially posh voice, and also a bit of a tongue on her.

Once she narrowly missed a train at the station.

—Shit.

The ticket lady stared at her.

—That's not very nice.

My mother stared back.

—Well, it's better than fuck isn't it?

My parents' speciality was the drunken, violent row. They used to regard a good row over a meal as a sort of art form, a theatrical performance, something to applaud.

Once halfway through dinner my mother picked up a fork, after some remark of my father's, and simply stabbed him in the face, ripping a bloody great hole in his nose.

Blood was pissing out all over the place. He insisted on walking out with the blood pouring down his face, rather than trying to staunch it in any way, and went home to his other family. A bit of a drama queen.

We carried on eating – there was nothing else to do. As I said, good training for the ambulance service.

Amir

Summer evening. A stabbing.

This being leafy, respectable suburbia, most times you get a stabbing, whether the perpetrator has done it to himself or someone else, it doesn't amount to much. Most times. But not tonight.

We're called to a male, thirties, multiple stab wounds, conscious and breathing.

Amir.

Well, that's interesting – the multiple thing for a start. On the way to the job we're told the assailant is his cousin – bloody hell. Attacker is still on scene, so we're told to hold back at the end of the road and wait for the police. It turns out the end of the road is almost directly outside the house.

When the police turn up it's just one constable who looks about ten years old and understandably nervous.

—Not going in there without backup, he says, and calls up on his radio.

So all three of us are waiting outside the house. I feel slightly absurd, but the fact the copper's shitting himself makes me feel better. Then out comes a woman in her late sixties or early seventies, nice and sort of mumsy-looking. She's not covered in blood or screaming or anything, and just looks at us with a resigned expression, raising her eyes to heaven. So I think sod it, let's go in.

In the front room the patient is a tall and skinny Asian man with long black hair, lying on the floor looking stunned. He's conscious and breathing, thank God. There are bloodstains all over his back. Another smaller man is bending over him, sobbing and saying sorry over and over again.

Then on the floor I see something which makes me think. It's a kitchen knife with blood all over it – the sort of thing the waiter brings you in an Italian restaurant if you order steak instead of pasta. About seven inches long with maybe a four-inch serrated blade. The blade is bent at an angle of about 30 degrees. Bloody hell. I've eaten with a knife like that at home – I know the sort of force needed to do that. The blade has hit a bone or something – flesh wouldn't do it. He must have meant it.

Anyway, he doesn't mean it any more. He's still sobbing and we practically have to drag him off the patient in order to get at him.

—They've always been at it, says the mum. Like cats and dogs, ever since they were kids.

I assess the patient quickly, and almost unbelievably, the damage doesn't look too bad. He's conscious and a good colour, the bleeding doesn't look too catastrophic from the outside, his lungs are clear and he can breathe well. Not for want of injuries. There are six or seven puncture wounds all around the back and abdomen, at least one over his lungs, and another where his heart would be. But his blood pressure's holding up and he's doing well. We get him on oxygen and into the ambulance as quickly as possible, while the policeman arrests the cousin, who is sitting on the sofa still sobbing how sorry he is. By this time the mum just looks bored.

We put in a call to the hospital and rush him in there – the danger is internal bleeding, and you won't know much about it until the patient's blood pressure collapses and he dies. He's fine all the way in, and I think he was lucky and made a full recovery, though we didn't find out. (We often don't.)

Nowadays Jo and I spend half our time at home listening to the kids shouting at each other and telling them to keep it down. This is a bit different. (They get on pretty well most of the rest of the time.)

Another time, at my parents' table, more training.

My mother's turn for treatment. She had cooked a huge risotto, which was on the table in a big saucepan. My mother said something which infuriated my father, so he got up, seized the handle of the pan, picked it up and smashed it over my mother's head. The risotto went flying out of the pan and splashed up against the wall.

My mother looked stunned. Now, of course, I would check her for concussion, injury, signs of raised intercranial pressure. But I wasn't that fussed at the time. (I was only about seven.) I didn't like risotto. I went down and got Kentucky Fried Chicken. No harm done.

Once my father came over, just back from abroad.

He'd brought my mother an enormous plate, beautifully patterned. The inevitable row began as he was leaving. My mother picked up the plate in front of him, and dropped it on the floor.

Smash.

Like miniature All Blacks, we had to hurl ourselves at him. We thought he was going to kill her.

Dave and Brian

Another 999 call. Mid-afternoon.

We're called to a dispute between two neighbours, which you wouldn't have thought was too much to worry about, but one of them's decided to settle it with a baseball bat.

When we get to the job, it's a nice detached house (though perhaps not detached enough) and the patient's sitting in his conservatory with blood pouring out of a couple of holes in his head, but he's still conscious and breathing, and not screaming in pain.

He and the neighbour have had some sort of argument over a borrowed lawnmower or something, and the neighbour's come round with the bat and seen if he'll take that in exchange.

And he's been pretty persuasive.

Our patient has at least two impact points on the skull from which the blood's coming, and at least four or five over his back when he fell to the ground and the neighbour kept hitting him. You can see the bruising. None of the wounds on his back are on the spine, so we don't have to immobilise him. Also, as much as we can judge, the skull around the head wounds seems to be intact (it takes a hell of a lot to break a skull). Even so, we're in a hurry to get him into hospital so the doctors can look at him.

Then the police turn up, not surprisingly. Just one girl on her own, small, blonde and pretty, who comes up to my chest.

We're sorting out the patient and she's taking down his particulars or whatever they call it when the wife looks over my shoulder.

—Oh my God!

—What?

—It's him! He's come back!

We look round and there he is, walking down the driveway towards us. Quite a big bloke.

Now I couldn't fight my way out of a wet paper bag, but I'm six foot two and I can see the poor police girl's going to struggle if he's serious. She's walking towards him undoing her handcuffs and thinking God knows what, so I fall in beside her.

Luckily, no such thoughts are in his mind. He's obviously gone home and thought about things and now he's walking towards us with his hands held out for the cuffs.

He comes quietly, as they say.

And we take off for the hospital with our patient, who's showing slightly worrying signs of getting sleepy, so we call it in so they're expecting us.

I didn't find out any more about the job, but I imagine relations in that street were pretty frosty for a while.

The past is a foreign country, they do things differently there …

At one point my father and stepfather met up in a cafe, two men together, having a summit meeting on what to 'do' about my mother, as if she was an outbreak of Ebola or a mad African dictator. My father asked my stepfather – still living with my mother – if he still loved her. If the answer was yes, he would break the affair off. The answer was no.

8

CHILDREN

The ambulance service often gives you a pretty jaundiced view of the human race. Especially when children are involved. That's when you get angry. At the parents, or fate, or whatever or whoever is in charge of this mess.

Louise

Called to a girl, bitten by a dog.

It's a grim, cold winter's evening and the address is on the outskirts of town, a small worker's cottage with the garden overflowing with toys and junk – not a good sign. Inside is mayhem. The house is dirty and untidy, but we're not too concerned with that because in the kitchen is Louise, with a bloody great hole in her face. The dog's somehow managed to bite her on the flesh of the cheek and ripped a three-inch hole right through the full thickness of the flesh to the jaw behind. Horrendous. She's in her aunt's arms and both are absolutely hysterical and covered in blood.

For some reason the police have been and gone. They've taken the dog with them. Some sort of bull terrier no doubt. Probably crossed with a tank or armoured personnel carrier. I don't know what they do with dogs in this situation but I imagine it's pretty terminal. Meanwhile we're trying to deal with the poor little patient.

We try to get a dressing onto her face to cover up the worst of it, and to give her some paracetamol, but it's fairly hopeless on both counts. She's screaming.

This is one of those jobs where there's little you can do apart from get them on board, make them as comfortable as possible, and go for the hospital, where they'll sedate the girl and get to work on her face. It's called 'load and go' in the ambulance service.

Load and go like fuck.

Just before we take little one and aunt in I go and tell

uncle what we're doing. He's a big, unshaven bloke who doesn't look too bright.

—I don't understand it. The dog's usually good as gold. But she's been winding it up all day. Mucking around.

—Winding it up?

—Yeah, pulling its tail and stuff. Winding it up. So we just left them in the front room together to get on with it.

Like I said, he doesn't look too bright. They just 'left them in the front room together to get on with it'. Which I suppose they have. Not exactly Barbara Woodhouse.

You really wonder with some people. You really fucking wonder.

At the station I tell Len all about it. He isn't impressed.

—Stupid buggers.

One night my parents went out to a party and left us to fend for ourselves. I was about ten. They were supposed to be back late, but didn't come back at all. Not until nine the following morning. They returned looking sheepish, with a pineapple as a peace offering. I still remember telling them a pineapple wouldn't have done much good if they'd been run over by a truck.

They nodded. All the loony parent stuff, the fighting and the drunkenness, was bound to have an effect. I ended up with psoriasis, anxiety and obsessive–compulsive disorder, unable to leave the house without checking the oven and taps are off a thousand times, that sort of thing. It's about feeling in control – and I suppose the service is all about being in control when everything's gone pear-shaped. I used to wait up in the evenings for my mum to get home, even if it was midnight or beyond, because I couldn't sleep knowing she was still out, frightened she'd come back and burn the house down drunk.

I'm all right now. Sort of.

Lucy and Jessica

Afternoon. We're called to a female, forties, unwell.

The address is a top-floor flat of a tower block in our area, and the patient's daughter's called us. She and her mother live together alone, she is only fourteen, and she pretty much looks after her mother, not the other way around.

The reason she looks after her mother is her mother is very, very fat. She weighs somewhere between 20 and 30 stone. She has a raft of medical conditions, some causing her weight gain, others caused by it. She sleeps in the front room because that's the only room big enough to accommodate her bed and commode, and it's almost impossible for her to walk anywhere. It's almost impossible for her to stand. She's enormous, sweaty, smelly – she's a human being, but for her daughter, she must be a nightmare.

Today she has an infection, one of many, and her daughter's called us because she can't be managed at home.

Getting her out proves almost impossible. We call another crew to help lift her across from her bed on to our carry chair, which can only just take the weight. We manage it, which is good, because otherwise it would be a job for the fire service.

I can't help thinking the real victim in all this, the person who's really suffering through no fault of her own, is the patient's daughter. She's a teenager – she should be going out and having fun, bringing friends back for tea and sleepovers, having boyfriends, being looked after herself. Instead she's a full-time carer for her own mother when she's not at school. I can't imagine she can bear to have friends back to witness what her mother's become, and you can just feel the horrific embarrassment she's feeling with us in the house. We treat her and her mum with as much gentleness and respect as we possibly can, for her sake, as much as her mum's.

But you feel your heart breaking when you look at her pale, shattered face.

Only about a mile away is another woman we go out to regularly. Again she's very large – at least 25 stone. She very rarely gets out of her oversize chair, even to go to the loo, but is hoisted by carers from the chair to her bed, then from her bed back to the chair. Her life is watching the telly. Jessica lives with her son, who is maybe in his twenties, and is also her carer.

He has his own bedroom in the flat, and lately if we arrive he sometimes doesn't even come out of it. Whether it's embarrassment, exhaustion or despair, who knows?

Tonight, as often, she's called us because she's having difficulty breathing. This is almost a chronic complaint – her lungs are being crushed by all the fat and don't function that well any more. She wants to go into hospital to be looked after. We bring our stretcher in and position it by her chair, but we have no training in how to use the hoist, and she would be simply impossible to lift, so we ask her to get up out of the chair and sit down on the stretcher. With enormous difficulty she manages it. Her backside has been crushed into the chair for so long it's become completely square, moulded by the leather. It's also covered in excrement from when she hasn't managed – or bothered – to get out and on to the commode.

Her son stays in his room – who would want to see this?

It's off to hospital we go.

Ambulance people, the NHS, the country as a whole, sometimes have slightly mixed feelings about people like this. There's confusion about the correct amount of sympathy in a situation that is sometimes, only sometimes, self-inflicted. The service has brought in special ambulances to deal with obese people – they were called bariatric trucks until somebody decided that was offensive, and now they're called something else. Crews often just call them fat trucks or the like now. And the stretcher on it – especially big – is called the 'Megasus' – it's written underneath it in large letters – which probably doesn't make the patients feel any better.

But it's the relatives I feel sorry for, especially the young girl looking after her mum and losing her childhood in the process.

Nobody seems to give a shit about offending her.

9

MENTAL ILLNESS

My parents weren't monsters, they had their own problems. My father's parents died when he was young, and then he'd had to go through the war, killing people and nearly killed himself. My mother grew up a triplet in a large family, stabbed in the head as a child by her own brother (no doubt accidentally) and neglected by her parents. Where does it ever end?

I suppose the beauty of it is – like in the Larkin poem – it never does. Your parents fuck you up but they were fucked up by theirs in turn. That's life, baby.

We do a lot of psychiatric calls. It's not something the NHS handles well, because it's so complicated and time-consuming – not like fixing a broken leg. From the ambulance point of view we're not much more than a taxi service. Maybe with a bit of amateur counselling thrown in.

But one thing the job teaches you is mental illness is just as bad as physical illness.

Alison

Called to a female, forties, cutting herself and generally having a meltdown. She has some history of self-harm and mental illness, and is staying with two friends in their flat. She's locked herself in the bathroom with the razor blades and is screaming and crying because her boyfriend's having an affair or left, I think. Worried friends have dialled 999.

Control comes over the radio.

— Police are towards but haven't given an ETA. Are you happy to approach with caution?

We are. Control does its best to shield us and assess whether a violent situation is dangerous, but sometimes it's difficult. Sometimes all the call-taker can do is ask the caller: are you dangerous? The caller doesn't often say: well funnily enough, yes – I'm a homicidal maniac, actually.

Anyway, we get to the address, which is the back entrance to a block of flats with shops round the front on the high street. One of the flatmates comes out to find us. The patient has gone ballistic and is screaming dire threats she'll kill them, herself, and everyone else besides if they call 999. Even though she's now sliced herself up with a razor blade and there's blood all over the floor of the flat. The flatmate's understandably nervous and upset. We're just getting a bit of info off her when out comes the patient.

She's about forty, with bare feet and weirdly bright green hair. Nice.

She's cut her wrists and ankles. All the cuts are a good three or four inches and deep, and now she's covered in blood. She's tried to cover the cuts with a rudimentary collection of tea towels and handkerchiefs, which aren't doing anything to stop the bleeding.

Quite a sight.

—Fuck you. I told you not to call!

She marches straight past us and her flatmate, screaming abuse, and out onto the main street with the traffic whizzing past. A bloke about her age has appeared from somewhere and tries to remonstrate with her a bit – the boyfriend – but when she approaches him he just runs away. We don't see him again.

She walks on up the hill, leaving a trail of blood behind her. I'm not too worried about her, more about what the sight of her would do to any young children passing by. She's lost a lot of blood, but she's still conscious and a good colour – she can't have cut anything fatal.

We follow her up the road, trying to persuade her to get in the ambulance, but she just screams at us to fuck off and carries on the threats against all and sundry. Then ahead of us the police turn up.

A PC and a WPC. They get out of the car a few yards ahead of her. It's pretty obvious, but I look at them and point out our patient just walking past them, covered in blood. The WPC reaches out to grab her arm and the patient goes mental.

She starts struggling, then whacking the WPC with all her strength, right in the face, again and again. We're all a bit surprised, to say the least. The PC and me jump towards the patient to pull her off the WPC, who has taken a couple of hefty blows in the face, and the PC sweeps her legs away and dumps her on the ground with her arms behind her back and kneels on her. She's still struggling as he tries to get the cuffs on her and the WPC leans in to spray her in the face with a pepper spray, but most of it misses because the WPC is crying with the shock and the fact she's taken a punch on the nose and can't see.

Eventually she's subdued, still screaming out threats and insults. The WPC is still sobbing slightly with the shock of it all, and motorists on the high street are staring at us sitting on this woman covered in blood and probably wondering why we all seem to be attacking her. Their eyes are about to pop out of their heads.

I think we need to get off the street somehow. Quickly.

The ambulance is around the corner, where I left it, so I run around to get it, then scream on blue lights the wrong way round the corner so we can get her on board and off the street.

Things begin to calm down, but only a bit. The PC's still kneeling on the patient's back, while we try to get some proper dressings on the horrendous cuts. She looks at the PC venomously.

—You fucking pervert. You're enjoying this, aren't you? Touching me up! Do you like it? Does it get you excited?

The PC looks anything but excited, kneeling on her back.

—Shut up.

He looks more concerned for his colleague, whose eyes are still watering from the punch on the nose. I lead her gently over to the ambulance and help her into it so she can sit somewhere quiet and out of the public gaze, and eventually more coppers turn up who help her colleague get the patient to her feet and into the ambulance onto the stretcher. One of them takes the WPC away.

All the way into hospital she keeps up a running commentary of filthy insults and accusations at the copper, calling him a rapist and paedophile and abuser, while he writes in his notebook and ignores her.

Only as we arrive at A&E does she relent, and collapses sobbing.

—I'm sorry. I didn't mean any of that. I'm sorry.

The PC still just looks bored.

—Whatever, darling. Whatever.

Barry

Hooray, we're off to the seaside.

But there's probably not going to be any deckchairs or ice cream on this trip. For a start, it's gone three in the morning. We've got a transfer of a patient from the local cardiac unit down to the coast where the big cardiology hospital is, going for an emergency procedure. The patient's nice and stable, no chest pain, it's a comfortable journey. No problem.

Or rather, none getting down there.

The problem isn't getting to this town. It's getting out of it. Even at five in the morning. At some point we've got to press the button on our truck telling control we're available, then hightail it out of town for the ninety-minute drive back to base, praying we're not spotted on the way. It's a bit like being a big juicy, tasty mouse, painted bright green and yellow, with a load of hungry eagles flying around.

We press the button and drive off out of the hospital, trying not to even breathe. Control pounces.

Male, forties, drowning incident, now fitting.

Fuck. And then fuck again. Drowning *and* fitting? What the hell does that mean? Surely if you're dead from drowning you can't be fitting? And if you're fitting you can't have drowned? Both jobs sound complicated. Together they sound like a nightmare.

Anyway, off we go. Apparently the patient's been fished out of the water by the coastguard and we're to meet their boat down on the beach. So access is going to be difficult, and we're going to need practically every bit of kit on the truck. Bollocks.

As always, life's a bit more complicated than that.

We scream down to the seafront, and take the obs kit, oxygen, drugs and the defibrillator with us. We'll have to come back for suction, the carry chair, stretcher and scoop, immobilisation stuff, a cuddly toy and the kitchen sink and anything else we might need.

I can see the coastguard rubber dinghy coming in the distance. Then as it draws near I see the worried-looking faces of the coastguard people, dressed in their red suits. They're staring at us as if to say: help! All I can see of the patient is a big pair of hairy white buttocks sticking up, thrashing around in the boat, as the patient's jeans have fallen down. Val stares horrified.

—What the fuck?

Behind us the critical-care paramedic is dragging another mountain of equipment down the beach as the dinghy hits the stones. Then the buttocks disappear and a face appears out of the bottom of the boat.

Barry.

It's not a face you'd forget easily. Barry's completely bald, and a lifetime of self-harming and dragging razor blades across his scalp has given him a whole series of ridge lines right across. Some of these have opened up and are pouring blood out down his face. He has wide staring eyes practically swivelling around, and the reason he has these is because Barry is, in non-medical parlance, raving fucking mad.

Nuts. Bonkers. Cuckoo. He's in the hospital several times a week, self-harming, overdosing, or just drinking himself unconscious. God knows what an actual diagnosis would say. Everything, probably.

He screams out to us, grinning.

—All right mate? Fucking great!

He steps straight out over the side of the boat and falls straight into the water in a heap of arms and legs and buttocks, then somehow manages to right himself and stagger out of the waves and on up the beach past us and towards the ambulance.

The critical-care paramedic knows him well.

—All right Barry? Why were you in the sea?

Barry marches straight past him too.

—Some cunt bet me I couldn't swim to France! I'll show him.

Barry's been drinking all night, indeed all decade, is not in the best of shape, and France is a good hundred miles away. But obviously in his crazy world, it seemed like a good idea at the time.

He marches on up to the ambulance and falls into it and onto the stretcher. We stagger after him with all our equipment, do some basic obs and put a dressing on his bleeding head, then take him up to the hospital. He's soaked to the skin and hypothermic, but otherwise seems untouched by his adventure. The critical-care paramedic smiles at us and gets back in his car and drives off, the coastguard boys just stare at us, before turning round and heading back out to sea.

Up at the hospital – practically Barry's second home – we get him on a bed and get some of his clothes off and cover him with blankets to warm him up. Within ten minutes he's bored with this and throws them off.

—Fuck it, I'm off.

—Barry, you really should stay here until you've warmed up a bit.

—Nah, fuck it.

And off he goes into the bright new day, staggering all over the shop with his jeans practically round his ankles. Legally I don't think we can stop him and I wouldn't like to try. I say a silent prayer no mother with her little children comes across him and his buttocks before he gets to wherever he's going. It's no sight for the faint-hearted.

10

UNSAFE DISCHARGES

Some people say their jobs are the best in the world, and George Clooney or David Beckham may have a point. But the ambulance service has a lot going for it. It's a varied life. Like a box of chocolates, you never know what you're going to get. I like working odd hours, with odd people. I love shift work, driving round town when everyone else is asleep and there's no traffic. I like being able to pick the kids up from school, and there's no better feeling than driving home on Monday morning knowing every other bugger is just starting their day. It's nice having a job where people are pleased to see you – I wouldn't want to be a tax inspector. It's nice being out and about, not pushing pieces of paper around a desk or something.

There are downsides to the job, obviously.

A Frenchman once said: hell is other people.

Wrong.

It's what comes out of them that's the problem.

* * *

We have a hamster at home. He's called Abdul, because he's a Syrian hamster and that sounded like a good Syrian name. (Bear with me a moment.)

He's very nice is Abdul. He sleeps all day and is up all night, making his wheel spin round or looking round his cage. He really likes peanuts as a special treat. He has some rather strange toilet habits though. He's very fastidious about where he urinates. We've bought him a special plastic box which he uses as a toilet, and he always pees in that, never anywhere else. And once he's peed he buries it in little granules, so it doesn't smell. All this is odd because his behaviour's very different when he opens his bowels. He does that in bed, keeping the stools in the bed with him and eating them again when he feels like it. All very strange, but he's a hamster after all. The reason I mention him is the other day we went out to a woman whose toilet habits are almost a mirror image of this.

Lisa

Called to a female, fifties, abdominal pain.

I haven't been out to this lady before, but many people have. She's an alcoholic and a frequent caller, with a variety of ailments and complaints. The flat is in a new development, and there's a sea of flowers in the front garden.

Unfortunately, the front room is a sea of empty wine bottles and overflowing ashtrays. The patient's slumped on the sofa while her lodger, looking slightly disgusted by the whole thing, is sitting halfway up the stairs.

Lisa tells me her stomach hurts, and so I sit down to ask some questions and take her pulse and blood pressure and suchlike. Judging by the evidence of drinking I have a fair idea of why her stomach might hurt, but I need to rule out other causes just in case.

—Does the pain go into your chest? (Could be a heart attack.)

—No.

—Does it go round to your kidneys? (Could be a kidney stone.)

—No.

—Does it go up into the right side of your chest under the ribs? (Could be gall bladder.)

—No.

—Have you opened your bowels recently? (Could be impaction.)

—Yes.

She has a slight temperature. Could be a urinary infection.

— Have you noticed your pee is very dark or smelly?

The patient stares at me blankly. Instead the lodger answers from halfway up the stairs.

— She wouldn't know.

— Eh?

— She wouldn't know. She doesn't go to the loo to pee. She just pees into the sofa. It sinks in.

— Oh. Right.

Oh dear. The same sofa I'm sitting on. It's a big, thick yellowy-brown affair, none too clean. Very absorbent. Could probably swallow gallons of the stuff.

Without making too much of a production of it, I get up and continue the assessment standing up. My bum doesn't feel dry for a long time. Val has to 'go out to the ambulance to collect something' quickly, doubled up with laughter.

And we take the patient into hospital, where she stays for only about an hour until she starts to sober up and decides to go home because that's where the wine is.

Ho hum.

This is the perennial problem with alcoholics. When they're ill and drunk, they want to go to hospital, but then when they sober up life's better again and they want out. And the alcohol's waiting. Everywhere.

The job was years ago now, just after we'd got Abdul. Then a couple of years after that, he got sick and began to swell up to an enormous size, the size of a cricket ball. Bilateral cysts in the stomach, the vet said, charging me three times what it cost to get him for the privilege. A few months after that he never woke up at all one morning, stayed lying in his bed, dead. I buried him in the front garden.

You should've let the children see his body, Jo said. It introduces them to death.

Fuck that, I thought. I didn't want to see it myself.

(Odd to see dead bodies nearly every week but end up crying over a hamster.)

If all human life is here, all human anatomy's coming up on the rails. You get to see people in the raw, and they're always fascinating. Sometimes seeing them in a rather more literal sense than God, or whoever is in charge of this mess, intended.

You see an awful lot of unpleasant substances in this job, not always coming out of the holes they should come out of. You need a strong stomach.

William

Many people in the service have pet hates: some don't do vomit, some don't do urine, some probably don't even like blood. Val doesn't really do faeces well. On some jobs if a patient has pooed themselves she'll go quiet and a certain look will come over her face – a bit like a hunted animal, eyes staring and panicking – and I know I need to step in because she's about to throw up. I'm quite good in this way and can deal with most things.

But today's different.

The day before yesterday we had the Station Wedding. Two colleagues who met in the service, tying the knot in a church up the road. It's been planned for months. Lovely. A marquee, people staying the night, that sort of thing. An ambulance-service bash, with colleagues behind the bar. I ended up throwing up and passing out on the train home – Jo isn't speaking to me, Val ended the evening being carried off the dance floor almost unconscious.

So we're still a little fragile.

We're called to an 85-year-old gentleman complaining of abdominal pain and constipation. The GP has been out and ordered us to come get him. The address is a pretty cottage in the countryside, and the patient is a pleasant and sprightly gent, but feeling sick and with the aforementioned painful stomach. It doesn't look too bloated, especially considering he's quite slim.

We assess William and do his observations, none of which are remarkable. It turns out he hasn't opened his bowels for a fortnight. We bring a carry chair in and move the patient out to the ambulance. Getting him on to and off the chair necessitates a little movement on his part, but within a few minutes we get him comfortable on the stretcher.

I'm in the back with the patient. I ask him if he's comfortable.

—I'm feeling sick.

He has gone a little pale.

Probably all that manhandling. I give him a cardboard sick bowl and get some tissue ready. We haven't even moved off yet. Then the patient throws up.

Someone being copiously sick when it's seven thirty on Sunday morning and you've not been long up yourself is not a great place to be, but this is worse. The patient's vomit is light brown in colour – the consistency of French mustard – and there's a lot of it. Bowls full. And it smells of exactly what it is – shit. Human faeces.

Among other very clever things, the human body is a container, for blood, urine, bile, food, liquids and so forth. The trouble is that if the exit for one – in this case faeces – is blocked, it's going to back up and back up and eventually come out of the entrance. Which is what's happening now. Our poor patient is vomiting up his own shit. And that's exactly what it smells like. The bowel is so completely blocked the faeces have backed up through it, up through his stomach, and are now coming out where the food went in days or weeks ago. I look on in horror but pat his shoulder and try to say reassuring things, then realise my own stomach is turning over and I'm very close to vomiting myself. I have to keep holding the bowl for him and wiping his mouth and therefore can't avoid looking at and smelling everything, and then unavoidably I retch and a bit of bile comes into my own mouth and I have to swallow it back down because I can't turn away. Val's in the front of the vehicle and is waiting for the signal to move off, but I can't give it because I'm swallowing my own vomit while inches away from a man vomiting up his own shit.

This is the life…

Val takes one look at what's going on and firmly slams the window between the saloon and the cab. The crisis passes after what seems an age. I get control of myself, and the flow of faeces from the poor patient's mouth begins to dry up with the third bowl filled. Eventually, he stops vomiting entirely and we're able to move off to hospital, where they'll fill him up with olive oil or operate to get his bowel working again.

And we're straight to the garage, to get some extra-strong mints.

Theresa

We're called to a female in a care home, eighties, 'inappropriate behaviour'.

It turns out the lady in question's a dementia sufferer, who's become too violent for the care home to handle. They've called us to transport her, well, anywhere, basically. The hospital first, then to a specialist nursing home which can handle her. However they do that.

Anyway, we roll up at the care home to find the job's been classified as a stroke, and so they've sent the nearest resource they can to stop the clock – Len. Len's got a student paramedic (learning on the job) in tow. Len doesn't get out to see patients much nowadays because he's an officer. They're trying to assess the patient and they're struggling.

Dementia's a diverse illness and can have diverse effects. There are probably almost as many symptoms as there are patients. Some go quiet and never say a word to anyone. Others regress to childhood, cuddling teddy bears and the like.

And some just get rude. World-class, Olympic-standard rude. A lifetime's suppressed aggression barges in the front door, inhibitions leave out the back, light the blue touchpaper and off we go.

Our patient today is a slim, well-dressed lady in her eighties. White hair, glasses, cardigan. Well spoken, well turned out. Quite the lady. But not quite the lady today.

Len and the student paramedic are trying to take her pulse and blood pressure and the like, but she's not having any of it. She glares at both of them with venomous hatred.

—Fuck off!

Len – ex-forces, remember – has a whispering, soft voice, slightly menacing and staring eyes. He looks at the lady as if he's deciding where to shoot her. (Mind you, he looks at most people like that.)

—Please darling, we just need to take a few observations, that's all.

—Fuck off and leave me alone! Cunt!

Len's experienced and he, like Val and me, has come across this sort of behaviour before, so he keeps well away. (Val once went out to a former nun with dementia and got slapped in the face for her trouble. The care worker took one in the balls.) But unfortunately, it's pretty well impossible to take someone's observations without touching them. Len reaches out to feel the lady's wrist for her pulse and she grabs him by the arm with all her strength and digs her nails in so hard she draws blood.

—Fuck off. Bastard!

He draws away nursing his arm. The student paramedic's not so experienced and not so lucky. He's kneeling at her feet – big mistake – trying to take her blood pressure. Finished with Len, our lady looks around the room at us with equally venomous hatred, then her gaze settles on the student at her feet. She says nothing.

He's looking down, not meeting her gaze, not sure what to do or say.

The patient looks at the student for a little while, expressionless, then sniffs as deeply and noisily as she can, and spits into his face.

Oh dear.

Bernard

We're called to an upmarket pizza restaurant in the high street. It could be a serious one. Male, sixties, hit by a bus.

Have the staff in the restaurant just seen it outside? Has the male been thrown into the restaurant by the impact? Or has he been carried in, barely conscious, head cushioned on a plate of garlic bread?

It's a busy Friday night in town, with loads of people out enjoying themselves, in and out of the restaurants and bars, having a good time. But the staff and customers of the chic Italian restaurant we arrive at are not having a nice time.

Our patient is sitting at a table by himself near the door, surrounded by lots of different bags. He's looking around at the other diners quite cheerfully, not obviously in any pain at all. Everyone else in the place is looking horrified. Absolutely horrified. The reason is our patient is very obviously living rough, but more than that, in well over a decade working for the ambulance service, he's the smelliest person I've ever come across.

The stink is really phenomenal, a composite of body odour, urine, excrement, unwashed skin and clothing and decomposing substances. It's enough to make your eyes water. And it's making everyone in the restaurant panic with a mixture of horror, revulsion and embarrassment. They're sitting over their pasta and linguine and this fellow's smiling at them and making them all want to throw up.

Apparently, he's just calmly walked into the restaurant and sat down, claiming to have been hit by a bus. So the restaurant's called 999 as fast as they can.

He's a big man in his sixties, with a massive beard with lots of things in it, a florid face, dressed in a huge collection of rancid, soiled garments. He has a huge booming voice, is quite well spoken, and doesn't appear to be drunk. He looks like a sort of Father Christmas living in a rubbish dump. And there's a certain sort of magnificence in him and the way he surveys the restaurant, totally unperturbed by the stink he's giving off or the looks shooting around the place. It's almost as if he's done it deliberately, just for a laugh.

Certainly there's no evidence he's been hit by anything, apart from the glares of horror and terror from the restaurant staff and customers. But the stink's unbearable, even for us, and we're used to it.

— Why don't we get you outside and onto the ambulance? The hospital's just up the road.

So he gets up quite happily and walks outside and on to the ambulance, and we take him for a very short trundle up the road.

The smell's so bad at the hospital I take the unprecedented step of leaving him outside while I go in and explain what's happened and what he claims has happened. He's a regular visitor. I get him a nice warm blanket and come out and cover him up in his chair and we leave him outside where a nurse will come out and see him. She might even bring him a cup of tea if he's lucky.

We're in and out of the hospital for the rest of the night. At first he falls asleep in the chair, and has a short doze.

Then about 1 o'clock in the morning he gets bored and gets up and wanders off.

The last I see is a collection of bags and a head bobbing off down the road happily.

11

LUCK

Afternoon.

We're in a leafy, quiet part of town on a nice spring day having a nice quiet shift. Birds are singing and old ladies are gently falling over not hurting themselves too much. It's all lovely.

Then, as often happens, it all goes tits-up.

Rita and Charlie

Called to a male, mid-twenties, back injury. Patient's a roofer, apparently, but there's nothing in the job notes that says anything about falling off the roof, so it doesn't sound too nasty – probably put his back out lifting some tiles. Another object lesson in ignoring the notes that come over on the computer – they are often wildly wrong. Chinese whispers: 'Send reinforcements we're going to advance' becomes 'Send three and fourpence we're going to a dance.'

As we draw up outside the house the controller comes over the radio.

—Could you take the dressings kit in with you?

Shit. No explanation as to why, but we're already thinking: uh oh.

The next minute or so is the bit that's really a nightmare. A man who looks like a builder ushers us around the side passage of the house pointing to another man kneeling on the ground clutching his back in pain.

—Don't worry about me, he says. They're round there.

He nods around the corner towards the garden. Around the corner we find the garden with a conservatory and a ladder leaning against the roof. Bricks and glass all over the place. There's a man sitting on the sofa in the conservatory with blood all over his head and arms. We're about to attend to him when we hear a child's screams from inside and he says the same thing.

—Don't worry about me. They're in there.

So we move past him into the rear dining room where a woman – his wife – is sitting on the sofa with a girl of about two who also has blood all over her head and arms. She's hysterical with pain and fear. Only then do we find out what's happened. The builders have been working on the roof – the couple have been looking after their daughter. Dad is on the way out with child alongside to ask if they want a cup of tea, at exactly the point the roofer is halfway up a ladder with a huge hod of bricks. He's lost his balance and dropped the lot.

The builder's fallen onto a retaining wall, but the pile of bricks has somehow smashed through the conservatory roof or windows, sending a shower of bricks and shards of glass down on the heads of Dad and child below.

A bit of a fucking nightmare.

My colleague runs to get the analgesic gas for Dad, while I try and get some pain-killing medicine into the screaming toddler and calm her down, which is not easy. I also get on the radio and scream for backup. Both Dad and toddler's heads, shoulders and backs are covered with a mass of cuts and blood, mixed in with bruises and brick dust and shards of glass – sorting it all out will be a job for surgeons. How neither of them are dead is a mystery.

Eventually, after what seems like a thousand years, backup arrives in the form of other crews and the helicopter doctor. Calpol hasn't helped the toddler much, and the doctor decides to sedate her before she goes to the hospital where she can be knocked out properly so the surgeons can begin repairing the damage. Dad goes in another ambulance. His head and shoulders look terrible. The builder is not too badly injured but God only knows what he's feeling.

It must have been a long and painful recovery for the three of them. All scarred for life. Just for a cup of tea.

A lot of life is about luck. Maybe all of it.

My parents were often lucky to get away with it.

My father used to spend his days writing articles about moral values and financial responsibility and that sort of thing. One night he came back to our flat so pissed he put the pressure cooker on to heat up some stew, then passed out on the sofa. The cooker blew up, the pressure cap smashing a hole in the ceiling of the kitchen. The hole was there for years afterwards.

He never even woke up. Just carried on snoring on the sofa.

He was a well-known and serious journalist who knew cabinet ministers and the like. Maybe the façade of respectability he had to exude in his working life led to a private life almost certifiable by contrast. He and my mother once visited a friend in Paris. A dinner party or something. My father ended up having a blazing row with a woman. She called him a motherfucker or something, objecting to his home life. I think he slapped her. She walked out and everyone else passed out. The woman went home and told her boyfriend, a bit of a hard bastard, who came round with a knife, intent on stabbing my father. But he couldn't get in, no one in the house heard him carving up the door outside – they were all unconscious.

Like *EastEnders*, but with posh people.

And lucky people.

I know I'm lucky too. Why am I rich and English, and he's starving and Ethiopian? Why have I kept it together and she hasn't? Why am I healthy, and they're ill? I sure as hell haven't had anything to do with it.

Is that why people believe in God? Because they can't believe it's just luck? Perhaps that's one of the lessons learnt from the service. I don't really believe in God, and one of the reasons is the randomness of life you see. You scream on blue lights to a man fallen off a ladder, but on the way you go past two people up ladders who haven't fallen off them yet. You scream on blue lights to a road accident, driving faster than you normally would, knowing more speed means more danger, no matter what training you've got, but you don't crash. You rush to a man who's suffered a stroke, but the fatter, unhealthier man you overtake gives you two fingers as you fly past because he's pissed off about the traffic or something.

A colleague from a different trust wrote a brilliant blog about the ambulance service, with a perfect title. *Random Acts of Reality*. You think of all this randomness sweeping all over the world and you think: What the fuck?

Victor

Some people don't recognise their own luck.

Night. Called out to a male, 20, rollover RTC (road traffic collision), head injury. The sort of call that gets the trauma junkies salivating. Cars that roll over do lots of damage to their occupants, throwing them around inside or sometimes out the window. Gory stuff. Off we go.

The patient is sitting by the road in the rain with a small graze to the top of his head. The car is upside down on a dual carriageway – a fast bit of road. He's taken it out for a spin, lost it on a bend, and… well, you know the rest. He's crawled out from the wreckage on his own. We go over his spine, his breathing, and all the rest as quick as we can, get him safely on the ambulance, then go over it again, much more slowly. Apart from the scratch on the head, can't find a thing wrong with him.

He's moaning about how pissed off he is. The car's very flash, brand new, and worth tens of thousands. This is more or less the first time he's taken her out for a spin and he's written her off. Then, to cap it all, the police come on board, breath-test him, and nick him for drunk driving. I'm beginning to feel a little sorry for him but then I step outside to look at the car.

It's one of those open-topped sports cars with no roof structure at all – just a little pop-up windscreen, now mashed to bits and crushed under the car. To a layman's eye it just looks like the upside-down car's had its roof and windows all ripped clean off. And then I start to think how the hell did he get out of this with just a scratch on the head? It's a bit of a miracle – we should have been shovelling his brains into a plastic bag by now. At the very least he should have broken his neck. I go back to the ambulance and as politely as possible tell him to shut up moaning. He's a lucky guy. Then we toddle off to the hospital.

The police will come down and get him later.

One of my parents' best efforts was in a Chinese restaurant – they were proud of this one. There were the usual insults and fighting, then one of them spat a mouthful of rice out at the other. The rice flew into one of those fans which restaurants and offices have, which then flung it all over the room and the other diners.

The restaurant manager loved every minute of it. He didn't ban them or anything. He asked when they were coming back so he could make sure he was there.

Lucky people.

Apparently Napoleon's advisers were once recommending a general to him before a battle, saying how good the general was at this or that or the other. Yes I know all that, said Napoleon. But is he *lucky*?

The trouble is, no matter how lucky you are, sooner or later it runs out.

Susanna

Morning.

An old joke: What do you give the man – or woman – who has everything? Penicillin. Ha bloody ha.

But the next job isn't funny.

I'm on my own on the car, with no Val to talk to, called to a female with breathing difficulties. The patient is paralysed from the arms down after a riding accident and also has a brain tumour which is killing her. That's all I know.

The house is like nothing I've ever seen. Rolling hills and woodland and deer wandering about. Down a long drive the road winds into a circle in front of the house, forming a parking bay with three or four spaces. A squillion's worth of shiny BMWs and Mercedes are out front. The patient's carer takes me into the house, which is a bit like a modern flat-roofed bungalow. Except modern bungalows don't have seven million bedrooms, a study, a library, a cinema and an indoor swimming pool next to the front room, which is twice the size of my flat. The whole place is sumptuous and enormous. Like a James Bond set. The kitchen is so huge I practically have to shout to the carer over the other side. Must be worth millions.

The patient's husband is there. The couple have a million children – there are pictures of them everywhere, all gorgeous.

This is the life.

And then there's the patient. A woman in her thirties. Gasping, overweight, and confined in her wheelchair.

Unable to wash or feed herself. She can talk and move her head and hands but that's about it. Her paralysis is so bad she can no longer move her chest muscles effectively and therefore can't breathe without help. She is slowly, inch by inch, minute by minute, being asphyxiated. There is a machine called a positive-pressure ventilation unit, which blows air into her lungs through either her nose or mouth to inflate them and keep her alive. She prefers the nasal cannula, which she has been using all day. As a result her nose has become inflamed and blocked up and she can hardly breathe at all now.

By changing her onto the mask which covers her whole face (and which she hates) some of the pressure is taken off her nose and she can breathe slightly more easily.

So: job done. But I can't help wondering what else to do for her – she's in such a desperate state. What on earth could the hospital do? Even getting her there would be a nightmare. Eventually I call out the doctor for want of anything better to do. The GP is a lovely man who arrives within the hour. Before he goes in we talk the case over. The GP knows it well – he's been caring for the patient for years – but he also knows the score. There's nothing to be done. The patient is nearly at the end of the road.

Basically, if she dies peacefully tonight of a chest infection, that would represent a good outcome, the GP says.

Jesus. When you put it like that it sounds stark, but that really is the way it is. It's torture, what she's going through physically, but it must be even worse seeing your beautiful house and family, knowing time is slipping away and ripping them from you.

I say goodbye but can't get the job out of my head. Didn't someone once say behind every great fortune there's a crime? But you wonder how anyone could deserve that.

I saw the GP some months later on a different job and asked after her.

No surprise what he said.

12

ROAD TRAFFIC COLLISIONS

The only time I've ever been a patient myself was one winter morning in 1994. I collided with a lamp post. I was riding my motorbike south out of London, in the outside lane. A brown Mercedes pulled out into the road from the left to join the traffic. It was morning and I had my headlight on, so I assumed it would pull out into the inside lane, but it pulled out straight in front of me. I braked sharply. There was a patch of diesel on the road which my front tyre hit.

The whole sensation was a bit like being blown up. You don't really know what's happened, except that something bad has happened, and you're suddenly not riding your bike, you're winded and wondering where you are.

Interesting, really.

The next thing I thought was: shit, I'm lying in the middle of the road in the morning rush hour, and I don't really want to be run over. I saw that there was grass behind me, so I picked myself up on two arms and one leg and threw myself back onto it. I only used one leg because the other one seemed numb. When I looked down at it, lying on my back, I could see that the shin bone was completely smashed, and the foot flapping uselessly below it like a dead bat as I held the leg up.

I thought: oh well, they can do amazing things with prosthetics nowadays. The next thought was: bloody hell that hurts. It was like having the worst case of cramp you've ever had, but being unable to do anything about it. All the time I was lying by the road with my leg hanging off a passing motorist knelt next to me, holding my hand. He didn't say much, just held my hand. It was amazing how much it meant. I never had the chance to thank him but I've never forgotten it.

Especially with the elderly, in pain or lost with dementia, sometimes just holding someone's hand makes a lot of difference. They don't always teach you things like that.

Susie, Jezz and Keira

Sunday morning. Called to an RTC, three patients, car versus house.

—House? asks Val.

—Yes, says the controller. House.

This is a little bit worrying. Houses don't usually drive down roads, so the car has travelled some way to meet one. Also, houses tend to be a bit stronger than cars, and can do them a lot of damage.

At the scene, we find a fair bit of carnage. The car's been driving round a smart new housing estate, left the road and driven straight into the front of a house, demolishing the wall below the front window. Inside a young mother is sitting shocked with her little baby at the end of the room which doesn't have a car poking into it. Both are thankfully unhurt, and the baby seems to think the whole thing is hilarious. Mum doesn't.

Outside the occupants of the car are three young girls. They're sisters, out for a drive. The driver's not complaining of any injury but her younger sister's got pain in the back of her neck. This is a big warning sign for us, so she's immobilised, which means fitting a cervical collar around her neck while someone holds her head, and then fitting her into a special mattress on the stretcher to keep her still until we can get her to hospital. There's no obvious injury to any of them, and we're not too concerned, but we've protocols to follow. Only a doctor, and an X-ray, can say for certain she hasn't broken her neck.

I'm more worried by the mental state of big sister Susie, who was driving. As we fit the collar to little sister and get her sorted out, big sis is looking at us with a look of frank terror on her face.

—What have I done?

I try to reassure her this is all precautionary and her sister will almost certainly be fine, but nothing I say seems to make any difference. No one in the house was hurt either, I tell her. Don't worry. Could have been worse.

She just stares at me, tears pouring down her face, terror-struck.

Eventually we get immobilised sister on to the ambulance and take the two other sisters with us. Immobilised sister is fine – all her observations are coming up roses – but elder sister is looking more and more distraught. Halfway to hospital she's almost gibbering with horror, sobbing, sniffling, staring around her wide-eyed.

—Look it's all right. She's going to be fine.

—You don't understand.

—What do you mean?

And it all comes out.

The three girls are pretty and smartly dressed and obviously not from the wrong side of town, so to speak, but they do look a little, well, young.

In fact they are a little young. Too young to drive.

Big sister has decided that, at seventeen and with only a provisional licence, it would be a good idea to borrow Mum's car without asking and take little sisters for a Sunday morning drive. And everything was going swimmingly until a dirty great house got in the way.

I begin to understand the look of terror on big sis's face. The car was, repeat was, a very nice saloon. Now it's a write-off stuck in a house. Little sister was a fit and active sixteen-year-old. Now she's lying immobilised on her way into hospital. Mum is not going to be pleased.

I do my best to reassure her, but in reality there's nothing much to say. Her Mum *is* going to turn up at the hospital and she *is* going to go mad and she *is* going to kill her – figuratively speaking. There's no way to dress this up. Her life is over.

Eventually, I fall back on the only thing I can think of to say.

—Nothing lasts for ever. Even this will pass.

I don't think it really registers. We get to the hospital and unload our patient and the doctors get busy making sure her spine isn't damaged (it wasn't). Big sister waits out in the corridor, staring into space, almost catatonic by now. I have a last go at saying the right thing, but she's unreachable, lost in a world of fear. We manage to get out of there before Mum arrives.

It wasn't going to be pretty.

I spent a year and a half ferrying people around in minibuses taking them in and out of hospital when I joined. It teaches you where the hospitals are, how to drive smoothly, how to talk to old, ill people, reassuring them life hasn't just reduced itself to pain and misery. Even when it often has. It's half the job. Then I did a two-month training course to move into A&E work and spent a year as a trainee.

You go from driving old minibuses to driving around in a £250,000 state-of-the-art ambulance. In the back, it mostly resembles a spaceship – the Shuttle or the International Space Station – lots of bright light and white plastic, lots of buttons and cupboards and equipment and machines lashed to the walls, a tiny escape window in the roof. There's equipment to help you deal with people who're having a baby, or have burnt themselves. People who're having a heart attack, or can't breathe. People who've broken long bones and short bones and all the others in between. There's equipment to help lift people who can't stand up, and equipment to help us manage people who won't sit down. There's dressings and splints and gloves in four sizes and drugs for everything from vomiting to pain relief to allergic reactions. And a cat, of course.

Eh?

The firm that makes the ambulances needed a little door for the rubbish bin on the side of the ambulance, around the size of a catflap door, so they went to a catflap door company, and bought a thousand doors. So the bin doors in all our state-of-the-art spaceship ambulances say things like *Pet Safe* or *Cat Flap* on them. Honestly. Many of our patients are quite confused before they even get in the ambulance. This doesn't help.

—Why is there a catflap in your ambulance?

—To let the cat in and out of course.

It says 'Biological Hazard' under the catflap, which probably fries their brains even more.

In quieter moments in the back of the truck with patients, I look at all the blinking lights and dials and machines and sometimes imagine myself in a spaceship, a million miles from Earth, warm and brightly lit but surrounded by a limitless void. Then the patient wakes up and vomits or something.

When I joined the service you did a week's training for patient-transport work, to learn how to drive smoothly, and then when you went front-line you did another two weeks learning how to drive fast on blue lights. The training's excellent and very thorough.

Only the service never calls it driving 'fast'.

I've always found this funny. As if they think the minute they tell you to drive fast you're going to floor it and plough straight into a bus-stop queue. They may be right. Instead they call it driving 'progressively'; making 'adequate progress' through the traffic or along the road. Maybe this is to take the excitement out of the whole thing, trying to weed out the nutters who just want to tear-arse around town making a lot of noise.

Like I said, they may be right.

The training emphasises that while they want you to get to the job quickly, they want you to get to the job. If you drive so fast you have an accident you're no bloody use to anyone, which is a fair point. Up to now I've done nearly a decade in the service without so much as a scratch, so I'm quite smug about the whole thing.

For eight years I drove on blue lights to jobs and never had an accident – some people had had hundreds.

Then I had a night shift…

Kolya and Paula

Tonight we sign on and fairly quickly get our first job of the night – eight-year-old boy, breathing difficulties. A Category A job – the most serious. And a kiddie. It's in the next town along the road, about ten miles away.

I'm driving and off we go.

All goes tremendously until we drop down the hill into the next town. At the bottom are traffic lights on red at a crossroads. I edge through these slowing down (you must treat red lights as a give-way junction and only go through if people let you) and can't see anyone coming. So I carry on through.

Then out of the corner of my eye I see a car coming through the lights to my right, still doing 30 mph or so, and not stopping. Smash! He drives straight into the side of the ambulance on my side, just behind where I'm sitting. The airbags in the car go off, and for a second it looks like the whole saloon of the car's just exploded.

—Gosh, I say. Or words to that effect.

Val tells me to shut up bellowing swear words and get out and look after them, while she gets on the radio to tell control what's happened. Now they'll need to find an ambulance for our original job and another one for us – we're off the road. The minute you have a crash you become a right royal pain in the arse.

Anyway, the couple in the car aren't too bad. They're a young couple from Eastern Europe, they've already got out of what remains of their car, and are really rather nice about

126

the whole thing. The driver's uninjured but his girlfriend has a nosebleed where the airbag's gone off in her face. I usher them into our ambulance, where at least they're safe and off the road, treat her nosebleed and check them over for any other damage.

The driver obligingly admits that as he was driving through the (green) lights he was looking in his mirrors at the car behind, which is being driven by a friend of his. They may have been racing each other or mucking about in a low-key way – this makes me feel better. The girlfriend's crying and I think the driver's frightened he's in trouble – maybe you get shot for this sort of thing where he comes from. I try to reassure them it's all right. Meantime I'm trying to stop my own heart hammering away and nursing a sore right knee. Eventually another ambulance takes them down to the hospital to be checked over, an officer comes out to see us, and we drive our truck to the station to do the paperwork. Other crews crowd around joyfully to have a look at the damage.

The paperwork takes about two thousand years. The ambulances are tracked by computer, which sends a signal every six seconds, saying what speed you're doing, whether you're on the brakes or the gas and other stuff. As I was slowing down into and through the lights, the last signal received before impact was 19 mph, braking. The officer reckons I was probably doing about 10 mph, which is judged fair enough. The very nice driver of the car saying he wasn't looking is also a big help. I had my blue lights on but didn't have the sirens on, but that's OK. You're not allowed to have them on if there are cars on a red light around you, as that may make them panic and push through the lights into someone's path.

So no blame for me.

The officer's really rather nice about it.

—It'd be better if you carry on with the shift, but I won't blame you if you go home.

Blimey.

The soft-soap treatment works. I put on a martyred expression, rub what's left of my knee and stagger out to the garage to carry on with the shift.

One evening my father fell off his motorbike and ended up in hospital. My mother heard about it and phoned her sister, who worked at the hospital. Her sister told her he was gravely injured and not expected to live. She went out and got rat-arsed. Then when she got to the hospital to visit him, she found him sitting up in bed, eating a boiled egg. She went ballistic.

Luck again. If life's a lottery, RTCs are even worse.

Kerry and Friends

About three in the morning. The lowest time of the night when you can barely stay awake – that time when you understand how effective sleep deprivation must be as a torture. Everything aches and you're constantly trying to keep your eyes open and feeling slightly sick. Don't know why they bother with waterboarding and the like.

Still – mustn't grumble. Back with Val.

We're called to an RTC down by the river outside town. Bad RTCs I find horrible, probably because I can remember how it feels. At night they are worse. It's dark, noisy, cold, frightening, and the stink of hot metal and spilled petrol is everywhere.

This one is bad. Five youngsters gone sideways into a wall. Someone saw them going past the ambulance station down the road, probably doing seventy or more.

The scene is like a vision of hell. Fire trucks are already there, so there is bright dazzling light. Bodies in the road, still in the car. Cold and noisy. One of the passengers (the lucky one) sits by the side of the road with his head in his hands.

Why was he the lucky one? No one will ever know.

We're the second ambulance on scene. The driver is badly injured but still alive, and a paramedic is looking after him. The female passenger beside him is dead already. Cans of stinking lager are all over the place.

Our patient is one of the back-seat passengers. The car has broken in half on impact with the wall and our girl is lying half in and half out of what remains of the back of it. She is unconscious. One arm is obviously broken, as is one leg. The other leg has been almost severed by the impact, and is only hanging on by a bit of muscle and tissue – a lost cause. We put her on oxygen, get a collar on her and set about packaging her up to get her into hospital. Both legs and the arm need to go into splints to keep them intact. We have to wait for the fire people to cut the door off because the bad leg is trapped between the door and frame, but eventually we manage it. At one point the patient starts to wake up and moans, so we do our best to reassure her and get a paramedic to put fluids up to try and maintain her blood pressure, which is collapsing with the blood loss.

Then it's on to the ambulance and off to the hospital.

As we leave the scene the fire crew are taking the roof off the car, with the driver still sitting there in the middle of what is left of it, the dead friend beside him. I heard later they left the dead friend in the car until the next morning – it was too complicated to get her out.

The hospital do their best for our patient, but it's no surprise to learn she died the following day – probably from internal injuries. Any impact that cuts a car into two halves 50 yards apart is not going to do your liver or spleen or anything else much good.

It was one of the worst RTCs I've been to. Three dead, the driver badly injured, and only the poor sod sitting by the side of the road relatively unhurt.

For years the wall just sat there, the damage repaired by the council months later, occasionally with flowers left by the families.

We rarely find out what happens to patients in the long term. But with some jobs you know they'll be scarred for life.

Physically or mentally.

If they survive at all.

Timothy

Being in the ambulance service is all about getting everything under control, and making sure things don't get worse, only better. With car crashes that's often hard to do. Before you can treat people, you've got to make sure the scene is safe, and no more accidents are going to happen. And then you've got to get the patient out of the car, which can take ages.

But despite the chaos and fear, some of them are funny...

Early Sunday morning, around 2 a.m. This is the sort of job I hate. Luckily I didn't do it but Val did. Her favourite-ever job.

Male, thirties, hit by car, high-speed impact.

Some people are 'trauma junkies' who like this sort of thing, and this one has loads of potential. The patient is probably drunk, and the road is a fast dual carriageway. Even on a misty Sunday morning the car could be doing 70-plus mph. And why the hell is the bloke wandering around on a dual carriageway at that time of the morning anyway?

They speed to the job fast, lights on, probably with dry mouths.

Things are a bit surreal from the start.

First impressions are horrendous. The car is slewed at an angle across the road, wrong way round, hazards on. The driver's standing beside it, staring, speechless. The bonnet of the car is crumpled and – worse – the windscreen is not just smashed but smashed to pieces. Most of it is on the road or in the car. Windscreens are not designed to do this.

The patient's been hurled onto the bonnet of the car and then right through the windscreen. He's ended up in the car itself.

Inside things get really weird.

Timothy's in his thirties, lying in the back of the car, covered in blood but still conscious, thank God. His left arm's smashed – open fracture above the elbow. There's blood coming from a wound above the right eye. He's smartly dressed, middle-class, very, very drunk.

The first thing to do is assess injuries and begin the process of immobilising him so they can get him to hospital to be X-rayed from top to bottom.

—OK, Timothy, try not to worry, Val says. We're going to get you out of here and off to hospital. You're doing really well. What's hurting?

—Nothing much. Arm's a bit sore.

Arm's a bit sore?

—Oh. OK. Well Timothy, we need to get this collar on you, to keep your neck still, and then sort your arm out.

—What?

—I said we need to get this collar on you, to keep your neck still, until we can X-ray it at hospital.

—Don't be ridiculous, I'm not going to hospital!

Eh?

—Timothy. You've been hit by a car at high speed. You've broken your arm.

Timothy looks outraged.

—Rubbish! I'm in a taxi. I just want it to take me home.

I don't need to go to hospital, there's nothing wrong with me.

—Timothy, you've been hit by a car at high speed. You're in it now. This isn't a taxi. Look at the windscreen. Look at your arm!

Timothy looks completely mystified.

—Are you sure?

—Yes, mate. You got to go to hospital.

—So this isn't a taxi?

—No. This is the car that has just run you down.

—Really?

—Yes. Really.

—Oh for God's sake. It's a waste of time. I'm fine. Never better.

—But you've broken your arm for a start.

—That? It's just a bit sore.

—No it's not. That's bone coming through. Look!

—Really?

It takes an age to persuade Timothy that he really has been in an accident, and then he keeps forgetting, whether through alcohol or concussion it's impossible to say. Eventually, with much persuasion that yes, this really is necessary, they get him packaged up and out of the car past the miraculously uninjured, and still speechless, driver.

God only knows what goes on in Timothy's brain at the best of times. Maybe he's a surrealist painter or something. On the way in to hospital he looks at Val as if a thought has just occurred to him.

—You're not by any chance Hungarian are you?

She's never been anywhere near Hungary.

He makes, as far as she is aware, a good recovery.
Back at the station Len shakes his head in wonder.
—Daft bugger.

13

SEX

—Doctor, I'm going blind.
   —Well, stop masturbating.
   —Why?
   —I'm trying to examine you.
   Sex.
   One of the reasons I like the job is you're dealing with life: living and dying, getting ill and recovering, breathing or not breathing. And having sex, of course. I'd been in the service a few years when the following job came in. But some jobs still make you wince.

Peter

Saturday night, Sunday morning. Things are not always as they seem.

It's always busy nowadays, but Saturday nights in this town are murder. Job after job, drunk after drunk. Exhausted. We are called to a male in his fifties in a less than salubrious part of town, complaining of a painful penis after sex.

A painful penis after sex? The correct medical reaction to this is: For fuck's sake! – call that an emergency?

And that's roughly what we think on the way to the job. We stop the ambulance and walk into the house, trying not to look disgusted.

Shows how wrong you can be.

The house is clean and tidy and pleasant for a start – ambulance people tend to be a bit judgemental – and the white-bearded man sitting on the sofa seems quite respectable. He appears sober, and looks very worried indeed. He is dressed in a T-shirt and baggy jogging bottoms.

—What's happened?

—Well, it's a bit difficult.

—Don't worry about that. Just tell us what happened.

—Well, my partner and I were making love when I heard a sort of snap.

—You heard a snap?

—Yes.

—*Heard* it?

—Yes.

Partner is a blond bloke – maybe thirtyish – standing in the corner of the room, looking startled. When we look at him he bolts out of the door.

—What do you mean, you heard a snap?

—Well I heard it snap, and then felt it go, and now this. It's sort of swollen. And it's gone blue. It doesn't look right.

I ask to have a look and he pulls the jogging bottoms down. His penis is the size of a large marrow and purple with engorged blood. It looks like a balloon filled with water that could burst at any second. I try not to gulp.

Basically, while pulling out and then pushing back in he has missed the target and hit the buffers, so to speak. The penis has bent and the stiffened tendon that runs under it which carries its major blood vessel has snapped. The flesh of the penis is filling with blood. There must be pints of it in there.

We're all sympathy now, making sure he's not suffering symptoms of shock at the blood loss as we get him gently on to the ambulance. We call the hospital to let them know we're coming in and what with, and I've never seen so many people in the resus department – the news must have spread like wildfire. What the man's done is unusual, and doctors love to see things like this. We gently get him onto a bed and I give the handover to the assembled scrum of onlookers. Then we wish him the very best of luck and leave to go and pick up the next drunk.

We never found out what happened to him, but I asked a doctor what could be done. The man would be catheterised with surgery to repair the tendon. But it would be a long and slow recovery.

*　*　*

Another row. This time my father walked out. I can remember my parents screaming at each other down the length of the communal stairs. It ended with my father yelling something about how the situation could not be changed. My mum yelled back:

—What do I get out of it?

My father stared up at her.

—My cock!

Eh?

My cock. That's what he said. I was only about six or seven. I didn't really know what he meant. Still don't know now.

(Not sure I want to either.)

Tania

Sometimes I think I may be a bit naïve. Thankfully.

Midnight. We're called to a female, fifties, with a leg injury, hit by a car. She's in a car park at the top of the motorway.

Seems like a nice place. The patient is lying on the ground, in obvious pain. She's wearing jeans, and when we cut them off there's obvious deformation, swelling and reddening to the right leg, just below the knee. It looks like a fracture. We get her on pain-killing gas as fast as possible and start to package her up to get her on the ambulance.

Seems like a very crowded place, this time of night. There are at least twenty or so people around, all sober and offering advice and trying to be helpful. The patient is a woman lorry-driver, parked up in the (smaller) car park just off the road for the night, and taking a walk in this one (presumably before going to bed in the back of her lorry) when she's been hit by a car. Strange. Whoever's inside is driving like a maniac trying to get out of the car park.

Everyone around is polite, sober, and remarkably well dressed. Most seem to be couples in their forties or fifties, the men smart and the women dressed in rather raunchy dresses. Lots of dyed blonde hair and cleavage. There are lots of smart 4x4s and pickup trucks here. The place is in the middle of nowhere, what can they be doing here? There are no nightclubs or bars for miles. The nearest place is the local university town, seven miles down the road. And it's midnight.

Anyway, we have other things on our mind.

We get the patient on to the ambulance, and luckily the gas is working well, taking some of the pain away. Since this is technically an RTC the police may turn up at some point, but we can't wait for them on a busy Saturday night – we need to get the patient to hospital, so off we go. It takes only a few minutes to get her into A&E, where we hand her over to the staff, who'll look after her. She'll probably have an operation tonight to set the leg.

Off we go to the next job. I don't think much more about it, except to mention it to the crew taking over our ambulance in the morning, as we prepare to go home, exhausted.

—There were just millions of people around. Weird. It's midnight on Saturday night, for God's sake.

—Yeah, well there would be.

Eh?

Turns out this site is famous as a 'dogging' site. I had no idea at the time, but 'dogging' is where different couples drive to a prearranged car park agreed by all. Then in their cars, some of the couples start to have sex, while other couples look at them through the window. Something like that anyway. Presumably some like to be watched, and others like to watch. Apparently you signify which you wish to be by some arrangement of headlights, or something.

Nice.

What's happened with our hapless lorry-driver is she's wandered past the wrong car, no doubt perfectly innocently. The couple inside definitely didn't want to be watched at whatever they were doing, and took off out of the car park like a scalded cat, running her down in the process.

Val is as surprised as I am. It doesn't make much difference to how the job went, but it's an education.

Sitting in his office back at the station Len laughs out loud.

—Dirty bastards.

All the loony parent stuff, wondering when they were going to stagger home or end up in an ambulance, was bound to have an effect. When I was about nine, I stopped getting undressed. I was frightened of having no clothes on. So I would wear the same clothes week in and week out, never taking them off, sleeping in a filthy polyester sleeping bag. This went on for some years. I must have stunk.

At university, I joined a scheme whereby in the holidays I would go to America to work for the summer. My father called an American friend, to see if he could get me a job for the period. He was embarrassed admitting to his illegitimate family. His friend wasn't. Maybe Americans are a bit less uptight about this sort of thing. And a bit more racist, maybe.

—What the hell you so embarrassed about, man? He's not *black*, is he?

(Charming.)

Funnily enough, as a kid, part of me was, sort of. I didn't wash much. I used to bunk off school on the days when we went swimming, so I didn't have to get undressed and show my filthy black toenails.

I still feel funny going into swimming pools now.

And saunas.

Chan

About 3 o'clock in the morning. Called to a male, forties, fallen down the stairs with a head injury. Off we go.

The location is a sauna in the town. There's a plain, rather drab front to the building, with the word sauna on it, and a picture of a young man smiling. All very nice. I've sometimes driven past and wondered what goes on there, but being an innocent and sheltered person, have never found out. (The missus and I once had a sauna on a camper-van trip to Finland at a campsite and it was lovely.)

Anyway, an unremarkable man in his thirties wearing a white T-shirt meets us at the front door and tells us access would be easier round the back. I'm not going to insult you by making a joke about this. Round the back we go, where he meets us and leads us inside. The sauna has many rooms and passages and fills the entire (huge) ground floor and basement of the building.

At first it's like a rather restrained and innocent nightclub, with red carpets and matt black walls, a few pictures of smiling young men dotted around, and a well-lit bar area selling sweets and chocolate bars. The only slightly odd thing is a large bowl on the bar, filled not with complimentary sweets but condoms.

Chan's a nice, polite, Chinese man on the darker floor below. He's drunk and has tripped and fallen down a flight of stairs, bashing his nose. We try to collar and board him but, embarrassed and drunk and claustrophobic, he'll have none of it. Eventually we decide it would do more harm than good, so we let him stand up and walk him out to the ambulance.

The route out is through the sauna proper, which is a huge darkly lit tiled area, steaming, with shower cubicles, a large jacuzzi-type pool bubbling away merrily, and more pictures of smiling young men on the walls – but this time they're all completely naked, and seem, to my fleeting glimpse, to be remarkably well endowed in the penis department.

There's a television high on one wall, but it's not showing *Coronation Street*. (Not unless *Coronation Street* has changed quite a lot since I used to watch it.) Val says she can hear noises going on in some of the darkly lit rooms off the main one, but we're quite busy and don't look. None of the shower cubicles have doors or curtains, and one completely naked man looks at us rather startled as we pass carrying our equipment. His is on display for all to see. Val's eyes bulge.

There's a sort of jeweller's shop cabinet with 'butt plugs' and 'cock rings' on display for sale. (Whatever the hell they are.)

On we go through the main sauna room. There are signs leading down a passage to something called The Glory Holes (another mystery). And finally in the sweltering steamy heat, the back door.

Outside we reach the fire escape. On it there's a notice. *Please Don't Have Sex On The Stairs.*

(Seems an odd thing to have to request.)

After this odyssey of mystery we finally get our patient on to the ambulance and settled. He's apologetic at all the fuss ('mortified') and we do our best to reassure him that we don't mind at all.

How could we? It's been fascinating.

I found out later what the 'Glory Holes' were.

(Trust me, you don't want to know…)

My parents' fights often seemed to be theatrical performances – exhibitionistic. They seemed to enjoy them. Once my mother bought me an air rifle for my birthday, and was keeping it under her bed until the big day. One night, they took their screaming row to bed. The next thing we heard was my father running out of the room, dressed only in his blue underpants, screaming to my eldest sister.

—Save me! Save me! She's gone berserk!

My mother came after him, clutching the air rifle. My big sister was visiting, home from university. She was studying theology. She wasn't home nearly enough for me.

I told Len about my parents one night when he was in a friendly mood.

—Bloody hell. They sound worse than the patients.

One thing you're going to come across if you do this job any length of time is the exhibitionists. People who really seem to like showing you stuff other people prefer to keep hidden. I'm not one myself so I don't really understand it, but it definitely happens.

Sometimes they're subtle about it. Sometimes not.

Ian

Val and I get a 999 call to a male, fifties, abdominal pain.

Despite having a filthy mouth and pretty filthy mind, Val also has a certain – somewhat misleading – air of sweet innocence about her. She is striking-looking, with perfect skin, full lips, prominent cheekbones and doll-like bright blue eyes. She's attending.

When we get to the job we've already been informed the patient is something of a frequent caller, and often goes into hospital with varying symptoms which are never fully explained but seem to resolve themselves. He's also missing a leg through diabetes.

It's the middle of the night, but the door to the house is open. The patient is on his own in the bedroom. He calls us through. The house is filthy and very smelly, with dirt and empty bottles everywhere. The patient is hugely fat, lying completely naked on top of the bed covers with his one leg spread to the side, his genitals glaring out at us. He doesn't appear to be in much discomfort but stares at Val fixedly, as if to say – there, what do you think of those?

It's not quite clear what she thinks, because she's staring fixedly at the wall, so I step forward and flick the corner of the dirty bedcovers up to cover the patient's modesty, but he's having none of it. He grabs them and throws them back again to reveal all.

I've got this pain here, he says, pointing to a spot about three inches from his penis. It's really painful. He's still staring fixedly at Val, not obviously in any pain at all, and she's

147

still studying the wall, so I sort of manoeuvre myself between them and take over doing the obs, trying to shield her from the appalling spectacle.

Needless to say they're all fine, so we persuade the patient to get some clothes on for the trip to hospital. By this time Val has fled to the ambulance to get the stretcher, and the patient watches her go with a disgruntled expression on his face.

And into the hospital we go. I go in the back.

At the hospital Fatima gives him one of her most ferocious stares.

He looks back, worried, and pulls the blankets up to his chest.

Unwell patient.

14

SUICIDE

The first experience I had of ambulance people was when I was about six. My mother told my father she'd taken an overdose during a row. He was furious, but probably thought he should do the right thing, so called 999. I still remember the looks the ambulance men gave us. And I still remember the mixed feelings I had. Fear my mum was dying, but also shame that strangers were seeing it. Whenever I go to overdoses now and there are kids staring up at me frightened, I remember what it was like and try and be friendly. I did one the other day. Mum had taken an overdose, Dad and four-year-old daughter were frightened. And it was Christmas Day. The overdose wasn't a serious one and wasn't likely to do much harm, so we had some time.

I ended up swinging little one round the room while she screamed with excitement, then blew her up an enormous balloon. We played catch with it in A&E. Hopefully she'll have some nice memories of that night.

(My mother hadn't taken the overdose after all. She just wanted my father to feel bad.)

Andy and Lorraine

A late summer's evening.

The call is to a female, fifties, suicide bid, in a neat little cottage in a neat little hamlet outside of town. When we get there we are let in by a man, also in his fifties or so, who looks at us glumly and leads us through to the neat front room where a trendy-looking woman wearing an orange suede skirt is sitting on the sofa writing in a notepad. She does not even look at us, just carries on writing. But it proves she is alert, conscious and breathing. The couple don't talk to each other and the atmosphere is charged with tension. They've had a row. Oops.

—What are you writing?

—A suicide note.

—Oh.

I ask the man to look around the house and pick up all the empty packets of pills she may have taken, before we go to hospital, and we take the lady's observations. The man comes back with handfuls of empty pill packets, including nasty stuff like paracetamol and tranquillisers.

—She's taken this lot, and I've taken this.

I stare at him.

—What?

—She's taken this lot, and I've taken these.

—*You've* taken that lot?

Bloody hell. My mind's racing. Val's staring. A double overdose! Do we call for a second ambulance? Will we need the police? What about the cat?

Since they are both wide awake, breathing OK, and happy to go to hospital, we decide we'll take them both in together – it will be quicker. But on the way in, it is the man who gives me more concern. His eyes are closing and he can barely stay awake. I have to keep shouting at him.

We get to the hospital without any mishap and hand the pair over to the staring Fatima.

She says nothing. Twice.

Two unwell patients.

Normally we wouldn't hear anything more about the job. Probably wouldn't give it a second thought.

Normally.

Three months later, I'm called to a doctor's surgery in the area, to a patient with chest pains. As we draw up the doctor comes out of the surgery to give a handover.

It is the same woman. The overdose.

(Don't know about you, but I never imagined doctors did that sort of thing. Shows how wrong you can be.)

I don't know if she recognises me but I sure as hell recognise her. I stare at her briefly, then get control. For the rest of the handover I look anywhere but into her face, in case she realises who I am. She doesn't appear to. We get the patient on board, all the time with me staring at the floor.

Afterwards Val stares at me.

—Wasn't that…?

—Yes. Yes it bloody well was.

Benny and Lyn

April is the cruellest month, apparently. But January runs it close.

Night shift.

It's midnight on a violent, stormy, freezing night lashed with wind and rain, and I'm on the car called to a male, newly homeless for the last week and not surprisingly, suicidal. Wants to jump in front of a train. Benny's a nice quiet lad, freezing and starving and soaked and miserable, but he's good as gold with me. Walks quietly over to the back of my nice warm car and gets in with no problem, happy to go to the hospital and not causing any fuss. Off we go. Apart from his lethally smelly feet, which are painful and swollen after a week of being cold and soaked, there's no medical concern. Maybe he's got trench foot.

All very routine.

Then halfway to hospital, as the heavens open again, we get to a long bridge over the river. Halfway over a car is stopped on the left, hazards on. On the right is a bunch of three or four people. As I slow and edge past, one of them flags me down desperately. I have a sinking feeling.

—Quick. There's a girl, threatening to jump.

For fuck's sake. I've got one in the car threatening to go under a train, and now another one jumping off a bridge.

I pull over to their side of the road and stop. I can't think what to say to my patient. *Guess what? You're not going to believe this…*

—Sorry about this. Just stay in the car would you?

He nods.

—OK.

I get out and get on the radio and ask for police as I approach.

It's a girl, about the same age as my patient, dressed in a hoody and standing on the wrong side of the railings on a ledge about a foot wide, one step from, well… you know. There's a couple on the sensible side of the railings, who've been trying to persuade her not to do it. She says nothing.

There are probably psychological protocols and techniques and stuff for dealing with this sort of situation, but I haven't a fucking clue what they are. I sidle up to her gently on one side with the bloke on the other and we have a bit of a chat. She doesn't say anything, but at least she isn't doing the don't-come-near-me bit.

Helpfully, it's pissing down.

She still doesn't say anything, and luckily doesn't do anything when I gently slip a hand around her upper arm so I have a hold of her. She's not big, so now even if she goes for it I've got a chance. The other bloke will help. And his girlfriend's being brilliant, chatting away quietly to her nine to the dozen. I look down. It's maybe twenty or thirty metres, and looks very cold and unfriendly down there. The river's at least a hundred feet across and flowing fast. If she goes in I'm not going after her.

Luckily, after a lot more chat we get hold of both her arms and she doesn't resist and I plead with her to come and sit in the nice warm car out of the rain. Benny's still in it with his smelly feet, thank God, and hasn't come out to join us on the ledge. They'd probably have lots to talk about.

Eventually she agrees, so we lift her up bodily, while the girlfriend grabs her legs, and lift her over. I'm not letting her go so she can climb over. That's when they always fall or jump. I know, I've seen it on the telly.

And we're back on the safe side of the railings, and after a short wait an ambulance and the police turn up to take her to the same hospital Benny and me are off to.

He's still sitting in the car good as gold when I get back soaked.

—Sorry about that, mate. Let's get you into the hospital. Off we go.

Later in the same crazy shift, I get called to another female, who might be suicidal or might not, the call-taker's not sure. She's not making much sense. She's called 111 and they've sent us to check her out. Because she's got a knife the police turn up as well. She has a lot of history, as it's called, with us and the police. She won't let us in but talks to us through the window.

—I didn't want an ambulance, I just wanted to speak to someone. Why are the police here?

—Well I think it's because you said you had a knife, love.

—Well I had the knife because I was chopping carrots.

—Oh.

—Anyway, I'm not suicidal and I don't need an ambulance, thank you very much.

—You sure?

—Yes.

—OK.

We leave her in peace.

Seems a bit strange – chopping carrots at four in the morning. The policewoman doesn't seem fazed.

—She should've used those small carrots. The little ones. They're nice and you don't have to chop them up.

Of course.

Off we all go.

15

MISTAKES

After my mother's overdose, I didn't come across ambulance people until one morning twenty or so years later when she died of a heart attack. She and I were living together with her house guest – cancer.

She'd been getting worse for nearly a year, on morphine and chemotherapy. I'd been living with her all that time, happy I was doing the right thing but secretly frustrated my life was slipping away. I used to have dreams she had died, then wake up disappointed when she hadn't. Then I'd have to deal with the guilt. I learnt that lots of people have mixed motives for the good (and bad) that they do. The important point is to do the right thing. The reasons why don't matter.

It was a Saturday morning and she died upstairs. She'd been getting iller and iller, but the end was still shocking and sudden. I suppose they always are. We called 999. I still remember giving her the kiss of life, retching with shock. The ambulance helicopter arrived and we left them to it. They came down a bit later and said it was no good – she was flat-lining.

I didn't know what that meant but it didn't sound good.

The local funeral company were on form. They sent two old men to pick up her body who must have been 150 years old between them. They couldn't lift her, so I had to give them a hand dragging her downstairs in a body bag.

Then they had an accident embalming her, and needed new clothes for the body. They lost her glasses, burnt the top of her coffin, then phoned up on the day of her funeral asking if they could drop her off at the house 'early'.

Brilliant.

But hey. We all make mistakes. Fifteen years in the ambulance service teaches you that.

Fifteen years also equals maybe 10,000 jobs done, maybe 20,000. They get better all the time. There's fewer and fewer times I come back and dive into my ambulance reference books, looking to see what I should have done, what mistakes I might have made.

—You haven't killed another one, have you?

Jo says it every time I look at the book. Ha ha.

—No, I haven't.

But not all jobs go smoothly, even if you know what you're doing. All you can say is you try and cope, whatever happens. Shit always happens.

Especially when you're just starting out.

Myra

I was still a trainee when I met Myra, working with an experienced colleague, thank goodness.

The ambulance service is all about making sure things get better, not worse. But when things go wrong, they go very wrong indeed.

Out in the countryside, afternoon.

Called to a female, sixties, cardiac arrest. We're not off to a great start because we are several miles away and it takes us hours to get there. Well, minutes anyway.

Too many of them.

We find a large Indian woman in the passenger seat of a car outside a bungalow, dead. Husband is indoors, still on the phone to us. They've been out to a film together, and as they've got back she's had a massive heart attack and died.

You haven't any seconds to lose, but the problem is you can't do effective resuscitation on a patient in a car. You need to be pushing hard down on a patient's chest for the cardiac compressions that push blood round the body to the brain to keep it alive. Impossible in a car – there's no room to move and you can't get at them. So we have to get Myra out.

That's the first trouble. She's a hefty woman. I pull her torso out sideways from the car as my colleague grabs her legs and we try to bodily lift her onto the stretcher. But she's a large lady and a dead weight and I don't have a proper hold of her. I'm no weakling but I can't hold her and she drops. I push my knees out to take some of the blow but it's no good. Her back and shoulders hit the pavement and her head hits the slab with a sickening thud. Just as her husband comes out of the house, sobbing and gasping. We grab her up again but there's already a smear of blood on the pavement and another on the sheet where her head finally ends up.

Great.

Never mind – she can't feel anything at the moment. Her husband can, though. His world is falling apart in front of his eyes. We try and reassure him and ask him to go back into the house to get her details while we get her into the ambulance and finally begin work on her.

It's not encouraging. She's in asystole, which means her heart is doing nothing, and she's been down ten minutes or more with no CPR. That's long past brain-damage time. Her brain's had no blood, so it's had no oxygen.

So it's dying. Or dead.

And things just get better and better.

By now another crew's arrived to help out, so with my crewmate and me in the back with the patient, one of the other crew drives our ambulance while the other drives theirs with the husband on board. We set off for the hospital in convoy. The route from here to A&E is quiet country roads and the bloke driving our truck doesn't know them. So we get lost. The husband being driven behind knows them only too well.

—This isn't the way to the hospital.

Great.

There's more. It's raining and we're pulling out from a T-junction with a learner driver – just qualified – heading towards us. In the gloom she doesn't see the blue lights, but the guy driving our ambulance thinks she does, so he pulls out on her. Crash.

She drives straight into the side of us at about 25 mph. I'm standing up in the back and go flying, head-butting my crewmate on the nose and then smacking my head on a cupboard. I've got blood coming from my head, and my crewmate's got it coming from his nose. The patient is oblivious, since she's dead. But that doesn't make it much better.

So we now have the fun job of unloading the patient, with one of us performing chest compressions on her, and wheeling her over to the other ambulance, in full view of the husband and the poor girl who's just qualified from driving school and bashed into us. She's no way of knowing we had a resus on board. All she knows is she's just crashed into an ambulance and next thing someone's being wheeled out of it dead.

After what seems like a thousand years, all this gets done and we get off to the hospital and deliver the patient. It takes about three minutes for the doctors there to decide there's no hope, and they call it and stop the resuscitation attempt, leaving the patient in peace. The family can come in and say goodbye. We do our best to commiserate with the poor husband, bitterly conscious what a bloody farce the whole thing must have looked.

Eventually someone arrives to make a better job of looking after him than we did and take him home. The patient goes off to the ~~morgue~~. mortuary.

And the poor girl in the car? Probably into a lunatic asylum.

Great.

When I was about six or seven, I was crossing the main road on my way back from school. A motorcyclist had come off his bike on the other side of the road and was surrounded by people. You couldn't see any blood or anything, but you could hear him moaning as he lay there. It made my knees weak and I wanted to go to the loo. So I ran off home.

Not long afterwards a group of us were coming home from school and came across a child our own age who'd fallen off his bike. His arm was all bent and deformed – it was obviously broken. There was an adult helping him. He looked up at us and told me to go off and phone an ambulance.

This was in the days when you had to find a phone box. I was scared of the responsibility and the attention and frightened I wouldn't know what to say, so I never called. I just ran off home.

I still feel guilty about it now. For all I know they're still waiting for the ambulance. Not a good response time. Not a good start to a career in the emergency ambulance service.

There used to be a T-shirt – *Love Means Never Having To Say You're Sorry*.

It's rubbish, of course. Not even death means that.

Most mistakes aren't serious, and you learn not to make them again.

But not all. After ten years in the job, with no complaints at all and a completely clean record, I made the worst mistake ever.

Jennifer

People ask what's the worst job you've ever done? Jennifer's the worst job I've ever done, by a country mile. But not in the way they mean. Len just looked at me sadly once we found out what had happened.

—Sorry mate. Can't help you much with this one.

Five o'clock in the morning.

Called to a female in her forties, complaining of a tingling down her right arm and pain at the top of her stomach. She's called the out-of-hours doctor service 111 and they've sent us because this sort of pain can sometimes be a heart attack. Off we go, through the 5-o'clock-in-the-morning mist and fog.

Cold. Dog-tired.

The house is a nice little cottage miles out in the sticks, very isolated.

The patient – in a dressing gown – meets us at the door and is a bit embarrassed we've come. She just wanted to speak to a doctor about her symptoms. She often gets the pain when she's anxious, and she's anxious tonight, she's on her own in the cottage (apart from a Jack Russell who looks like he wouldn't say boo to a goose), and she's had a stressful week at work.

We follow her into the nice sitting room, sit her down, and have a good look at her. Everything seems absolutely fine. The pain's gone and the tingling in her arm is easing too. She thinks it's all just anxiety and we're inclined to agree. All her clinical observations are fine: blood pressure, pulse, temperature and blood sugar, and the basic ECG we do on her heart looks fine too.

So we have a nice chat about her life and work. She's a lawyer by trade, very interesting to talk to. She decides that, no thank you, she won't come to the hospital with us that night. If the symptoms come back she'll either call back or speak to the GP in the morning. She's a nice lady and we think we've done a good job calming her anxiety. After another brief chat we say a friendly goodbye, wish her a peaceful night, and leave. She seems perfectly comfortable and we have no worries about her at all. Tickety boo.

It becomes the worst job I've ever done about two days later, when her daughter comes round and finds her upstairs in bed.

Dead.

She calls another ambulance but there's nothing they can do – she's stone-cold gone. At some point between when we left her and when her daughter came round she went up to bed, lay down, and quietly died. No signs of any vomiting or thrashing around, no blood, nothing. She's just lying peacefully in bed, dead. The post-mortem says a heart attack.

And so begins an inquiry that takes over a year and leads to my crewmate that night sobbing before a disciplinary hearing and she and I being found guilty of gross misconduct and receiving a one-year final written warning, threatened with dismissal from a job we love. We should have done a more in-depth ECG, should have discussed things with the clinical desk at HQ, should have driven faster to the job (though it's difficult to know what difference that would have made).

The bottom line is, somehow, we should have known she was going to die and got her to hospital, where they might have saved her. But we didn't, and so she died.

Sometimes the job is hard.

We didn't think she needed to go to hospital, didn't think anything was wrong with her at all, and I can remember signing on at the start of the shift and hearing over the radio that the hospital was rammed and we should try 'alternative pathways' for our patients, if at all possible. I don't think death counts as an 'alternative pathway'. I went and saw her daughter afterwards and said sorry to her face, trying to explain what we'd done and why we'd done it. She was very nice about it and gave us tea and biscuits and said she understood.

But her mum's still dead.

Even after years in the job – and plenty of people have done twice what I have – you learn that you can only do your best, follow the protocols and give some people the best chance you can. Some things just aren't meant to be.

16

HEROES

Sometimes it goes right. Even when it goes wrong. Just like on the telly.

Jed

We are called to a male, late teens, breathing difficulties.

The trouble with the service's system of call-taking is that almost anybody can have breathing difficulties. They can have them because they're too busy throwing up after fifteen pints. They can have them because they're sobbing their heart out now their girlfriend's left them.

Anyway, luckily we're just around the corner, and when we get to the job, nobody at the house seems that worried.

—He's upstairs, Dad says. He just came in from the garden and said his asthma's playing up. Dad looks more mystified than anything else.

Upstairs in the bedroom the patient is a boy of about seventeen, lying on the floor unconscious and already very nearly dead. He is still trying to breathe, so every second or so his torso spasms with the unconscious effort, but absolutely nothing is going into his lungs. They are locked shut. He's blue and his oxygen saturation level is 62 per cent. It should be 100 per cent. He's going to die in the next few minutes.

We immediately put an oxygen mask on him – not that that will do much good – and I run for the drugs bag. He needs a shot of adrenalin to keep his heart going and gas to open his lungs, and he needs it now. I give him the injection and we bundle him onto a chair and carry him downstairs and out to the truck.

And of course the fucking tail-lift on the ambulance decides that on this one fucking job it is going to pack up.

Nothing. It's jammed and won't go up or down.

Fucking whoops.

We don't even have time to call up another truck – they'd never get here in time. So we carry him around to the side door and lift him through, which is almost impossible up steep steps with a totally inert body. I'm sweating buckets by now, as is Val. We get him on the bed and I set up a piece of equipment that allows me to force gas into his lungs which may free them up and get them working again. We do this for perhaps a minute and his oxygen levels come up into the low 90s but he's still unconscious. We don't even have time to deal with the family, who've watched what's happening dumbstruck.

—It's a life-threatening asthma attack, is all I tell them. See you at the hospital.

Then we go screaming off.

On the way in his oxygen levels are staying in the 90s with us breathing for him, but he's still unconscious, and once at the hospital they have further drugs and steroids that will also get his lungs working again. We hand him over and they get busy.

Then we can breathe again ourselves. We go out to clean up the truck and do the paperwork and make a cup of tea, and about twenty minutes later I go back into the resuscitation bay to see how things are going. He's sitting up in bed, bright as a button, surrounded by his family. Clearly has no idea what's happened to him. The family's looking quite relieved, but I'm not sure they quite know either.

Anyway, we just saved his life, and it doesn't happen all that often.

We say goodbye, wish them all well, and tell them we never want to see him again.

Outside, Val looks at me.

—Now *that* was a good job.

Back at the station, a bit pumped up, we tell Len.

—We saved his life, even with the ambulance trying to kill him!

(You learn in the ambulance service there's no such thing as an inanimate object.)

He nods at us, frowns, and walks off.

—Make sure you get that tail-lift fixed.

17

TIMING

Mankind cannot bear very much reality, as the poet said.

Because of this, and because paperwork is taking over, the medical profession is chock-full of acronyms. It saves time. CCP for central chest pain, SOB for shortness of breath, C?C for collapse query cause. You get the picture – there are loads.

But there are more exotic ones.

One morning we're called to David, a forty-year-old student asked to get off the bus on the not unreasonable grounds he has no ticket. The bus inspectors turn up to order him off. David collapses with agonising back and leg pain and breathing difficulties, so they call 999. The medical acronym for this is LOB, or Load of Bollocks. Others include TUBE, for Totally Unnecessary Breast Examination (apparently) and NIN for Normal in Norwich (if you're in Norwich, I suppose). One of my favourites is DFKDFC – Don't Fucking Know, Don't Fucking Care.

(Obviously we would never dream of using any of these.)

And then there's TF BUNDY. You don't want to see that written on your medical notes – not on your nelly.

TF BUNDY – Totally Fucked But Unfortunately Not Dead Yet.

My father had a massive stroke in 1995 which destroyed his brain and turned him into a vegetable. I'd only really made a relationship with him in the last ten years as I'd grown up myself. He was a famously witty and talented man, a great talker and drinker, despite the 'complications' mentioned, and then within seconds he was reduced to lying in bed, staring straight ahead, feeling and saying nothing. He was fed by a tube going into his stomach. He went on like this for eighteen months. We ended up having conversations with his doctor and nurses about whether treatment or even food should be withdrawn and he should be allowed to die. It was an emotional minefield and caused terrible suffering. Eventually a chest infection killed him.

He already had two families that we knew of. But he'd also worked out in West Africa for a time. At the funeral we were wondering if a third one might turn up?

He'd collapsed at Swindon station after a lively lunch and was taken by ambulance to the nearest A&E and then on to the John Radcliffe, where they operated on him to keep him alive.

I'm not a brain surgeon and I don't know the ins and outs of it, but I can't help wondering why. When you have a stroke they scan your brain to see where the stroke is and what damage has been done, and it must have been obvious the damage was massive – my father wasn't going to recover. Would it have been better to let him go? It made me think about the doctors and surgeons, or perhaps to be fair the legal framework in which they now operate. I'm sure they thought they were doing the right thing, but I wonder.

Still. What do I know?

Dawn

Most doctors are wonderful, with a warm and comforting bedside manner that does wonders for their patient's peace of mind, at a time when they're frightened, ill and vulnerable.

Others – just a few – can be abysmal.

Early morning.

One of the most common calls we get – to an 85-year-old female with chest pains.

At the house the patient's doctor is already there with her, which is unusual, and has called us. She is lovely, with a warm bedside manner that is massively comforting for the patient. She knows the patient well, has been out to her many times, and even came out this morning. Most doctors, hearing the words 'chest pains', order you to put the phone down and redial 999 immediately, thereby washing their hands of the whole affair. With perfect justification, of course.

But not this one. She gives us a brief handover.

The patient is an anxious and frail old lady, who nevertheless lives independently on her own, looking after herself. She was recently widowed. Her symptoms are classic for a heart attack – chest pain radiating into the left arm and jaw, dizziness and nausea, the works. When we wire her up to the ECG machine there is little room for doubt – it's a myocardial infarction. A stonking great heart attack.

Now comes the tricky bit. We have to get her out into the ambulance and down to the hospital as fast as possible, while at the same time being as reassuring and gentle as possible and looking like we're not rushing at all and don't have a care in the world, so that her heart isn't put under any more strain. It's a fine line.

At the hospital we take her into the resuscitation room, which if you're not used to it is probably terrifying – starkly lit, lots of busy nurses and doctors flying around, strange machines and equipment. And if you're unlucky, someone moaning or screaming in the bed next to you with only a curtain between.

This is when you have to be even more gentle and reassuring to the patient, and we try to be, as our lady is obviously terrified. The nurses strip her to the waist to do another ECG. Three A&E doctors come in to discuss her ECG and treatment. The bald facts of the matter are they must decide what sort of treatment to give her and whether it's worth giving it to her. They don't want to put her through needless suffering, or waste treatment on someone who has little quality of life or is going to die anyway. The doctors stand at the bottom of the bed, staring at her, firing questions. They haven't introduced themselves. She sits there, naked from the waist up, covered in wires, terrified.

—Do you own your own home?

—Do you get out much?

—Do you see much of your friends?

—Do you do your own shopping?

Our lady is now confused and baffled as well. No one makes any attempt to cover her up, so I go back to the bed with a blanket to keep her warm and try and reassure her. Then I answer some of the doctors' questions for her, making sure I give the right answers, since she – thank God – doesn't realise these shouted questions might decide her fate.

After a while the doctors make a decision and thankfully bugger off, leaving the patient to be cared for by the nurses. Once I have handed her over we say goodbye and leave, furious.

Barry and Meg

There's no question you get immunised to suffering in this job, you see so much of it. But some jobs are just *sad*.

Called to a male, suicide attempt. The location is a comfortable house in a middle-class town. When we get there a woman's waiting calmly for us outside the house.

—He's in there, she says, pointing inside. She looks lost.

When we go in we find at the back of the house a kitchen, and in the centre of it a man – her husband. On the table in front of him is a letter.

The man is dead – has been for some time. He's grey, has no pulse, and his body temperature has already dropped a couple of degrees. When we wire him up there's nothing – he's gone.

The woman's by now in the room with us, so we say how sorry we are – there's nothing we can do.

—That's all right, she says. I knew he was dead. I waited half an hour before I even called you. I just wanted to say goodbye.

It turns out her husband suffered from an incurable and terminal disease. He's wanted to take his own life for years. This is something like his third serious attempt, and he's succeeded. He's taken a hefty overdose. Wife had only gone out to do the shopping, then come back to find him gone.

The letter is just too sad to read.

He's in a better place now. Hopefully.

There's little we can do. Because it's an unexpected death the police will attend as a matter of routine, and luckily there's a family friend who comes round to sit with the bereaved. A long and painful road has come to an end.

After a little while we leave and, apart from how sad it is, think little more about the job.

Only later do we find out there's a postscript.

The inquest decides – I won't go into the details – he couldn't have done it on his own. The wife is charged with helping him. Only six months or a year later is she (and perhaps he) allowed to rest. We hear from the newspaper she pleads guilty. She's given the minimum sentence the judge can legally give.

Hopefully both of them are at peace now.

Callum

Summer's afternoon.

It's been a quiet shift knocking about leafy suburbia, then we get called to a male, twenties, cardiac and respiratory arrest.

—*Twenties?* says Val, Jesus Christ.

Unfortunately, he's probably not going to help.

Male patient with terminal illness, young kids and a wife. The couple used to live abroad but came back to England when the husband got sick. Parents also present. A real family party.

The reason they're all there is the doctor's been out and told the patient this is it. It's Saturday afternoon and he's unlikely to see the weekend out – the illness is too far gone. The nurses have been helping out – they're at the house too. And the doctor's proved right. The patient's gone and died.

The problem is they've called an ambulance. We're forced by our own protocols to try to reverse the cardiac arrest, no matter how hopeless, if we've got there within a certain time. Otherwise we'd be breaking the law. Only if there's a specific, signed, doctor's order can we do nothing, and there isn't one here.

About as rubbish a situation as you can walk into.

The house is a nice pleasant one – most are around here – and the patient's in the first-floor bedroom. We rush up the stairs with our equipment. The parents are downstairs sobbing. The kids – thank Christ – are nowhere to be seen, and the wife and nurses are upstairs with the patient. He's lying on the bed, with red hair and big eyes, but the illness has wasted him.

The nurses look up at us like we're about to attack him.

—Please don't do anything! Please don't do anything!

—What do you mean?

I can see he's not breathing and there's no pulse. By now we should be dragging him off the bed on to the floor to begin resuscitation. You can't do it properly on a bed.

The nurses are pleading with us.

—Don't do anything! It's hopeless. The doctor said he won't last the weekend. All you'll be doing is prolonging his misery!

In my head I couldn't agree more. God knows he's suffered enough and I can see it's hopeless. He's obviously gone. But I'm also thinking: why did you call us? If you'd left it twenty minutes we could have left him alone. As it is we're legally obliged to do something.

I don't want to do this.

I start doing chest compressions, to keep his circulation going, but stop short of dragging him off the bed. I'm trying to think of what's best to do, but I also don't want to end up in court and on the dole in the same week.

—Can you get the doctor on the phone? Quick!

I carry on doing gentle chest compressions on the bed, trying not to disturb him too much. He's so thin and wasted that proper ones would break every rib in his body. I carry on with one hand as the nurse hands me the phone. Doing CPR on the telephone. Ridiculous. I explain our protocols to the doctor as quickly as I can, still doing compressions. He gets it immediately.

—How can I help?

—Will you order me to stop the resuscitation now? Over the phone?

The doctor agrees.

—Yes. Right. I'm ordering you to stop. Stop it now. I'll come round immediately and sign your paperwork.

And so thank God we can leave the poor man to rest in peace with his family, instead of breaking his ribs and dragging him off to the hospital to be declared dead in some shitty anonymous resuscitation room. We take our equipment off the bed and some calm descends, but we're not out of the woods yet.

You should never outlive your children.

His poor mum, waiting downstairs, doesn't understand why we're stopping. She's furious at the doctor for telling him he'd never last the weekend, and believes that's triggered him to give up. She may be right.

Her husband and the nurses try to make her understand that if it wasn't today it would be tomorrow, and if not then the day after. But none of it sinks in. We try and say the right thing, but what the fuck can you say?

We pack up our stuff and go.

18

BODIES

After I gave up journalism I spent years in the removals trade, humping furniture. That was quite like ambulance work as well, seeing people in their raw state. Divorces were usually the worst, when you were carrying out the furniture to two different trucks, trying not to bump into the warring couple. Not always the worst. Once we turned up to a job and an elderly lady came to the door, looking rather shocked.

—Morning! Ready for your move, love?

—He's dead!

—Eh?

The lady's husband had fallen down the stairs that morning, and died. The ambulance had been out to him but there was nothing they could do, so they had left him where he'd fallen. The police would come presently, to rule out foul play, then the undertakers would come to pick up the body, which was lying in a heap at the bottom of the stairs.

Removals companies get booked up months in advance.

—Well, look, that's terrible. We'll go.

—No you bloody well won't. I've had you booked months in advance, and we're moving today. You'll just have to work around him.

And believe it or not, that's exactly what we did. Stepping over the body on the way up the stairs and stepping over it on the way down with the beds and furniture. After about an hour the undertakers turned up to take him away. We tried our best but we still stepped on him a few times. At the time I'd never seen a dead body before – it was something to think about.

Not any more.

Georgie

It's a warm summer's evening, and a bunch of us are sitting around in the crew room of the station, just started the night shift, putting the world to rights.

Unfortunately, the weather doesn't extend to Len's mood. He marches into the crew room in a filthy temper, takes all the unwashed crockery in the kitchen and dumps it in the bin, then insists we sweep up the leaves out of the garage outside. The garage is the size of a football field. Everyone groans inwardly. Val rolls her eyes. Luckily, just as someone goes to get the brooms from the broom cupboard our beepers go off. We have a job.

International airport.

On the way the call comes over the radio – not always a good sign – and the controller sounds confused.

—Got a job coming in at the airport on an inbound flight.

—Roger?

—Well, if you could just go and assess.

—What?

—Well it's a female, terminal-illness patient. She's… er… coming in with her family.

—What's wrong?

—She's… Well, she's dead.

—Eh?

—Erm, she's sort of… dead. Died sometime on the flight.

—Well, what do you want us to do about it?

—Well… erm…

The controller can't think of anything else to say.

185

—Just go and assess her, will you? Assess.

Great, says Val. What does he mean? Assess her? If you're dead you're dead.

Ours not to reason why. We shoot off.

The plane hasn't landed yet, so we wait on the tarmac of the runway for it to make its deafening entrance. Then the doors are flung open and we make our way down the aisle to the patient, trying not to bang the passengers' heads with the airway bag like the stewardess does with a guitar on *Airplane*.

The patient is sitting with an oxygen mask on between a man of her own age and a young woman. Luckily they are at the very back of the plane, so the other passengers can get off. The patient is cold, stiff, dead.

I put a foot in it straight away.

—Do you know the lady?

—Course I fucking do. She's my mum.

Val gives me one of her looks. *Brilliant. Fantastic. Well done.*

—Oh, sorry. Erm… well, we have to do a few checks and so forth, just a formality you understand. Perhaps you'd like to get out of your seat?

The daughter and her father – obviously still shocked – get up and are escorted by the stewardesses away down the plane. Other family members behind go with them. The patient is a terminal-illness patient, coming back from a 'goodbye' holiday with her family. Father and daughter had a short nap on the plane, and she, sadly, took the chance to start a longer one.

The problem we have is the plane is a public place, and more to the point probably due to fly out in an hour or so, so we have to get her off and down to the mortuary. Getting her out of her seat and into the carry chair and down to the ambulance is no problem. The illness has wasted her and she's frozen with rigor mortis into a sitting position anyway. But when we lie her on the stretcher her legs won't go down, so she lies with them drawn up grotesquely. The husband stays with us while we wait on the tarmac for almost two hours for the port authority doctor to come and certify death. Then it's off to the morgue at the hospital in the dead of night.

The mortuary attendant looks like death himself as we wheel the patient in. The mortuary is freezing – not surprisingly – and has what looks like oversize grey filing cabinets all along the walls. In one section there are tiny little filing cabinets standing alone. I can hardly bear to look at those.

—Just pop her in this one, the attendant says, opening the drawer.

It's still like a filing cabinet inside, just wider and a good six feet long. But not very deep. We lift the patient in and lay her gently on her back. But the cabinet won't close, because her knees are still drawn up in the sitting position. When we try to close the drawer they just bang against the top. We look at the attendant in panic.

—No problem, he says tiredly.

He steps forward and tucks the patient's knees down and under the top lip of the drawer, then lets them go and pushes the head down to fit that under and in as he shuts the door.

Jesus, we're thinking. Now she'll be jammed in there – you won't be able to get her out! When you open the door, the back of her head won't come out.

—No problem, says the attendant.

He reads our minds.

—It's the rigor mortis. She's stiff as a board now but she'll be floppy as a baby by morning.

—Oh right, we say. Of course.

We get the fuck out of there as fast as we can.

Michael

Freezing midwinter afternoon.

I'm on my own in the response car today and the next call is a bit odd.

Man in car. Apparently dead.

The location is a parking bay, a hundred yards from a big house converted into flats.

The car in question is a knackered old Vauxhall with the windows a bit steamed up. It's a murky afternoon and I can hardly see into the car. I can just make out, lying across the back seats, almost buried under various types of bedding and duvets and wearing a woolly hat, a man who does indeed look rather dead. He doesn't appear to be breathing, his face has the waxy yellowish colour skin has when the blood has gone, and even when I bang loudly on the car window his eyes don't open.

Unfortunately, there is something else in the car that is definitely not dead – a large dog that looks like a Staffordshire bull terrier. Every time I bang on the window the dog snarls and barks ferociously.

Normally I'm pretty good with dogs, but I can see this is not a good situation. The dog's in its home space. God knows how long it's been there or how hungry it is, and its owner is lying in the same car, dead. Now a weirdo stranger is trying to break into the car to attack both of them, and the dog's going mental. I try to open the door a fraction (it's not locked) and the thing goes ballistic. I shut the door again.

189

I get on the radio and ask for a police dog handler to come. I'm not going anywhere near the bloody thing. The patient looks very much like he's past helping anyway.

Within a few minutes the policeman arrives and I explain the situation to him – the ferocious dog, the corpse, etc. The copper doesn't look too cowed. He goes back to his car and gets a handful of biscuits from a packet he keeps for his own dog, then opens the door and holds out a biscuit for the savage dog. The ferocious beast takes the biscuit gratefully, starts eating it, and jumps down peacefully with his tail wagging and totters off to the field nearby, where he proceeds to do the most enormous poo imaginable.

The copper gives me the same sort of look Val sometimes gives me.

Plonker.

The poor thing must have been desperate.

Anyway, I can get inside and double-check the man really is dead, which he is. He's stiff as a board, so much so that the undertakers are going to have a nightmare just getting him out of the car. He's a big bloke. There's no signs of suicide or foul play and, thank God, no signs that the dog – now busy stuffing biscuits down its throat as fast as it can get them – has started to eat him.

But he's obviously been in there some time.

One of the residents of the house has come out to see what all the fuss is about and knows the deceased. The dead man was a friend of his, and was working on his car two days ago, but then vanished, leaving his own car here. He has a flat locally, has had some mental health issues in the past, and makes a living working on people's cars. He's been known to sleep in his own one before now.

—I thought he'd just gone home, says the resident. He looks devastated. Didn't realise he'd been out here all bloody night.

It seems the patient's worked on the car into the night in the freezing cold, then decided to go to bed in his own car with the dog, probably with a drink or two on board. Trouble is the temperature two nights ago was minus ten (it's not much warmer now), and even with all the bedding and stuff, he's frozen to death in the car. Death by hypothermia can be like that. Your heart just slows down and you feel more and more tired. And then you suddenly start to feel quite mellow and warm and cosy – and that's it. Not a bad way to go.

He's been in the car anything between twenty-four and thirty-six hours, and it's a shock for the residents of the house, most of whom knew him. He's been lying in the car dead and they've been merrily driving in and out of the place all day, oblivious.

To cap it all, the poor dog's got a large tear in its scrotum, which looks horrendously painful but doesn't seem to stop him being rather sweet and good-natured about the whole thing, provided the biscuits keep coming. The copper promises to take it off to the vet to get it seen to, and then it'll go off to the pound, hopefully to find another owner. Having not eaten the bloke's face off and not even had a poo in the car, I can't help thinking it deserves a bit of luck.

I say goodbye and leave, as there's little for me to do. The undertakers will come for the body in one of those private ambulances used to carry dead people in, and the police will deal with the dog and the car. And the residents will go back to their nice warm homes and fires, feeling just a little shameful, though you can't really blame them, it's not their fault. Not every car has a dead body in it...

...though some do.

Like the one that had a dead body – presumably the owner – in it, but also a sticker from the council on the windscreen, saying they were going to remove the car soon if it wasn't moved. The sticker was days old.

(Who they expected to move it I don't know.)

19

THOSE LEFT BEHIND

We lived in a flat in a house in south London. We used to play with the kids from the flats next door. Three of the kids were from an Egyptian family – their father was a film director or something. One day he got in his car, drove to the seaside, drank a bottle of vodka, and cut his wrists. They never talked about it.

The trouble with our job is you aren't just treating the patient – you're also treating their family. Sometimes the treatment for one is unbearable for the other to watch. Sometimes it scars them for life. And there's nothing you can do about it.

Roger

Before we got together, Val did a night's overtime with a colleague. Even more foolish, they did it on a Saturday night, in a town near here that's a bit lively, to say the least. Lots of drugs, lots of drunks, lots of headaches. They had a typically busy Saturday night shift with plenty of the above. Then, about four in the morning when elsewhere things might quieten down, they get the job from hell.

It starts as a male, forties, fallen down the stairs.

So far, nothing too unusual, even with the age. Probably drunk again. When they get to the job it is a typical location, big Georgian house divided into flats. Very nice. The flat they are going to has a front door on the first floor. Behind it is a flight of stairs to the flat on the floor above. There's a woman screaming behind the door but she's not opening it.

—Can you open the door?

—No! I don't know where the keys are.

For some reason the flat doesn't have a Yale lock, only a Chubb one. And the woman inside – hysterical – can't find the keys.

—He's fallen down the stairs – help him!

—You need to go back up and look for the keys. We can't help if we can't get in!

Eventually they manage to calm her down enough to get her to go and find the keys and – miracle of miracles – open the door.

Then it gets even worse. The patient is a big man, naked,

who has fallen down the stairs from top to bottom. He's broken his neck and is in cardiac arrest.

Shit.

They've got to start cardiopulmonary resuscitation on him, doing chest compressions and getting air into his lungs, in a tiny cramped square at the bottom of the stairs behind the door, while trying to get a collar on him and immobilising his neck and head just in case there's a miracle and his spinal cord is still intact. All in order to get him off to hospital. All the while the woman who's called the ambulance – realising from what's going on that the worst has happened, goes ape-shit. As Val said, to steal from Jeremy Clarkson, it's a bit like doing the *Times* crossword while being eaten by a polar bear. They try and calm the woman down by asking her to jot down some of the patient's details – give her something to do. Name, next of kin, that sort of thing. It often helps, but not tonight.

—I don't know any of his details! I only met him two hours ago! He's called Roger!

Shit.

It turns out they just met in a club tonight, and have come back to Roger's for, well… you know. Possibly a bit drunk. It's Roger's flat. He's got up during the night to go for a pee and fallen down the stairs and broken his bloody neck.

In any dates-from-hell competition this has got to be right up there.

Somehow they manage to get Roger out into the hallway where they can work on him, carry on the resus, then with the help of another crew get him down the stairs and into the ambulance. Then it's off to hospital. Val never found out what happened to Roger but it's not likely to have been a good outcome.

As for his new friend…

Tracy

Early Sunday morning. The 999 call is to a female, fifteen, with abdominal pain. The call has been classed as Category C, so it's not the most urgent we deal with. And it's the first job of the morning, to a girl with a tummy ache, so we trundle off down to the location at a fairly leisurely pace.

Halfway down we get a call on the radio. The family have called back and could we get a move on? It's still just a fifteen-year-old with abdo pain. Curious, but we put the blue lights on anyway and speed up.

When we get to the location it's a fairly standard house in one of the better parts of town (there aren't many). There's a south-east Asian-looking man in his fifties outside, at the front door, staring at us. He looks deeply shocked. He points up the stairs.

—She's up there.

He makes no attempt to come with us, just stares into space. Even more curious. At the top of the stairs we are greeted by a woman in her fifties, also looking absolutely stunned.

(You've probably already guessed.)

Inside the bedroom is the teenager – their daughter – and she's definitely got abdo pain because she's having a baby. And I don't mean pregnant, I mean having a baby. Fearsome contractions, waters have broken. Urge to push and crowning. All the signs. It's not going to be long. We settle her down and get her on the pain-killing gas, and ascertain there is probably still just about time to get her into hospital. So we get her on board.

—Who's coming with us? I ask the parents.

They are staring at each other, still in shock.

—You go, says the man.

So Mum climbs aboard and we tear off up to the hospital. In between sorting our girl out I am wondering if the parents can seriously not have known. The girl is quite slim. No matter how many jumpers and Demis Roussos dresses she wore, surely it must have been obvious?

Anyway, what do I know? We are just in time and get her to the hospital about five minutes before she gives birth to a nice healthy baby. By this time both parents are standing in the corridor outside still looking like they've just seen Elvis.

Then ten minutes later along the corridor comes another couple in their forties or fifties, also looking absolutely stunned. Between them they are accompanying – maybe frog-marching – a gormless-looking youth of about seventeen or so. Lanky long hair and spots, jeans practically around his ankles, Kevin and Perry to the life.

The two couples look at each other with staring, questioning eyes filled with rage, mystification and panic. You can see it all there.

Then, after we have said a very delicate and unsmiling goodbye and gone down to the ambulance to clean up, out of the hospital comes the gormless lad, still looking mystified, but quite cheerful. He looks around at the bright new dawn and then down at his phone and starts texting someone.

We can't help but smile. Maybe he's texting God to get him out of this one, but it doesn't look like God's replying today. I can't help feeling a twinge of sympathy as we drive off and wave goodbye. If only he knew.

Like I said, often it's not the patient you're treating, it's the family.

Philip

Wednesday, morning.

The call is a Category A Red 1 – the most serious. To an elderly male in cardiac and respiratory arrest. Dead, in other words.

We scream to the location, trying to get there as soon as possible. The flat is up on the third floor – no bloody lift – with the door open and the patient sitting on the sofa – no pulse and not breathing. He'd dropped his wife off at the garden centre to buy roses that morning, then come home to do some errands and died on the sofa. She'd found him like this.

Since we don't know how long he's been down we have to assume there's still a chance. We pull him on to the floor and begin cardiopulmonary resuscitation.

Resuses are always full-on, and you tend to focus on what you're doing and ignore everything else. It's busy.

After about fifteen minutes we begin to give up hope. The patient is not responding to drugs in his system and his heart is still showing no activity on the monitor.

It is then that you finally take in your surroundings. The patient is a tall distinguished-looking black man with snow white hair. I notice there are two video boxes on the floor by him, even though the television is off. They would have been at the patient's feet when he was sitting on the sofa. From the covers of the boxes it is very obvious what they are. The one I can see shows a lady doing something to another lady and neither have much in the way of clothes on.

200

Hard-core porn. Bollocks.

As if life wasn't complicated enough, now we have to deal with this. He's come back from dropping his wife off (to buy roses!) and... well, you know.

We have to try and protect the wife. Maybe she never noticed. In between chest compressions I get the two video boxes and push them as far as I can under the sofa.

The man's daughter arrives presently. By this time we have given up on the resuscitation – there's no hope. I gently ask her if I can have a word in private outside.

—What is it?

I'm trying to think of the best way of putting it, but they don't teach you this in training school.

—Sorry to mention this, but we were thinking of your mum.

—What do you mean?

—It would appear your dad may have been looking at some... er... gentlemen's videos... when it... er... happened. So to speak. We've hidden them under the sofa.

—*Gentlemen's videos?*

What the hell else can I call them?

—Yes.

The daughter looks tired and weary and sad.

—Oh, that. Yeah, she told me on the phone. Don't worry – she knows. I'll get rid of them later.

As we go back into the sitting room she looks at Dad fondly and gives a sad laugh.

—Bloody hell, you old bugger. What are you like?

It might not have been dignified. But maybe that doesn't really matter any more.

20

PILLARS OF THE COMMUNITY

It's nice being in the ambulance service. You're respected, liked, admired.

A pillar of the community, someone trusted and responsible. Like doctors.

Aren't you?

Oscar

Evening. Called out to an RTC, one patient, eighties, injuries unknown.

Road accidents can be all or nothing. There are a lot of fast A roads round here which seem to be where the most serious ones occur – cars heading towards each other at high speed with no crash barrier to keep them separate like on a motorway.

Anyway, luckily this is a nothing one. An elderly gent driving back from the golf club, clipped by another car going the other way too fast and which hasn't even stopped. Probably driven by 'youths'. Our old boy has been taken into someone's house for shelter and so there we check him out but he's not injured, thankfully. And it looks like it wasn't even his fault.

He's a lovely old boy, very sprightly and apologetic at all the fuss, and grateful. Everyone loves him.

Problem is, when the coppers arrive and breathalyse him he blows positive – over the limit. It turns out he might have had one or two dry sherries down at the club and they haven't quite worn off.

The copper's an old friend of mine (his family looked after Abdul the hamster a few years back while we were on holiday, although this isn't strictly relevant), and I know he's a nice bloke and I can see in his eyes that he really, *really* doesn't want to have to nick this sweet old man when it wasn't even his fault.

But the old man's blown positive. The limit is 35, I think,

but he's blown 37. Millisomethings of alcohol in the breath or whatever it is.

—What I'll do is just go out and see if there are any witnesses, then we'll try again, shall we? the copper says.

He's got a certain leeway because the local police don't prosecute unless you blow over 40, or something like that. Between 35 and 40 you're still drink-driving but you just get a caution.

But when he comes back in the old boy blows 39. The copper's looking desperate now. The readings are going in the wrong direction. At this rate the patient might even blow 40 next time and have to be arrested. Everyone would hate that.

Especially the copper.

—I'm just going to have a look at the damage to the car, then we'll try one last time, he says.

He looks at me as if to say: *Do something*. Val does too.

And so I have an idea. While he's out of the room I get the old man to hyperventilate as hard as he can without feeling dizzy, breathing in and out as deeply as possible, cleaning out his lungs.

Val's laughing.

He's still doing it when the copper comes back five minutes later, so I quickly signal him to stop before the copper sees what we're doing.

And bingo, he blows 33. We can all relax. Daughter has turned up, and can take lovely old Dad home, the copper doesn't have to nick him, and we can go back to base. Everyone's happy.

Technically we've aided and abetted a crime. And let me emphasise this isn't ambulance service policy. Or mine, most of the time. But I haven't lost much sleep over it.

Emily

Evening.

Kidnapping is defined as the unlawful taking or transportation of a person against their will, usually to hold them unlawfully. Either for ransom or in furtherance of another crime, or child custody or whatever. If asked, no doubt, most lawyers will tell you it is 'a bad thing'.

In the ambulance service the answer is: some days yes, some days no.

We're getting towards the end of shift and called to a female, seventies, unknown problem. We're working out of a station very near the hospital, but the call is nearly fifteen miles away. By the time we get there, we have about an hour of the shift left, and we're forty minutes' drive back to the station and hospital through the traffic.

So.

When we get into the house it's to find a slightly unusual patient – a woman in her seventies or so, quite respectable house, quite respectable-looking lady. Only, this evening she's drunk. Wandering around the front room in her knickers bumping into things, very unsteady. Once we've sat her down and done her obs we can rule out all the other worries that might be making her behave like this. Besides, the smell of booze is overwhelming and the empty bottles are all around the kitchen.

Val looks at me and whispers.

—She's wankered. Pissed as a fart.

We phone the daughter.

She says it's a recurring problem. Mum gets sozzled, then phones 999 and says nothing. Just attention-seeking, I suppose. The police have got fed up with her and so now they're palming her off on us. But the daughter doesn't want to come over – she's been over enough times already.

—Just put her to bed and leave her. She'll be fine.

And that's what my crewmate and I are thinking of doing, when an evil thought occurs to us. Val gives me one of her meaningful looks. If we leave her at home, we'll have to press the 'available' button on the ambulance, and like as not get another job, and we've only got another forty minutes left of shift. The job could be anywhere, we could be hours late off. If, on the other hand, we take her to hospital, by the time we've got there and handed her over we'll be about five minutes from the end of our shift, and very close to the station.

Not exactly a 'two-pipe problem' as Sherlock used to say.

She doesn't want to go, and her daughter doesn't want her to go, but strictly speaking, she's not safe to be left alone. She's stumbling all over the place and knocking the furniture about. Me and Val look at each other, but no words are really necessary. We both know the score.

Unlike the patient, who doesn't really understand how she's suddenly been manoeuvred into a carry chair and hustled out to the ambulance. We phone the daughter back and tell her, and she bows to our superior judgement, probably just glad someone else is dealing with it. And off we go to hospital.

Fatima isn't exactly chuffed to see her, but needs must and all that.

Patient safety must always come first.

21

WONDERFUL PEOPLE

Hell is other people – but heaven is too.

It wasn't all doom and gloom with my parents – they were quite a laugh a lot of the time. And ultimately, it's far from doom and gloom in this job either. You meet some of the most extraordinary people you could ever hope to come across.

Vikram

The ambulance service is a wonderful institution and the best job in the world, as I have often said, but sometimes it reminds me of the old cliché about the swan, gliding serenely about on the surface, paddling away furiously underneath. With the service, it's paddling with only one leg – the other's fallen off.

I jest of course.

The next patient's a bit like that. Male, thirties, breathing difficulties. A fairly average job, nothing remarkable. The man lives in a fairly average part of town, in an average street, average cars in the road, fairly average bungalow.

But this man's not average.

When we get to the job we let ourselves in using the key safe as the patient apparently can't get to the door. Inside is, you guessed it, pretty average, but very neat and tidy, spick and span.

Our man is in the front room, sitting in a wheelchair with an oxygen mask on his face. There's the whoosh of compressed gas being released under pressure from a machine on the floor, and the tubing runs from that machine to the mask on his face. He doesn't look too distressed.

In fact he looks calm as anything.

Through the mask he tells us the story. He's paralysed from the armpits down. His head, arms and shoulders work – nothing else. An accident. Because the abdominal and chest muscles that expand and contract the chest and fill the lungs don't work, he can't breathe. The machine is what's called PPV – positive pressure ventilation. It blows air into his lungs under pressure using the mask, which inflates them so they can do their work. Without it, he'd be dead in minutes.

He has two machines, one which services the front room and kitchen, and one for the bathroom and bedroom. Why he can't have one hanging on the back of his chair all the time I don't know – presumably there's a reason. He plugs the mask into whichever one he's closest to. And the one that does the bedroom and bathroom is broken. Which also means if the one he's on now should pack up, he is dead.

That's what I call a breathing difficulty.

Now we're here we could take over his breathing for him if that one packs up too, but even so, he's astonishingly cheerful about the whole thing. He can't call the company to fix the machine because they can't hear a word he says. So he's pressed his care alarm button and – would you believe it? – apologises for wasting our time!

We reassure him it's quite all right and phone the company for him and they will be round in a jiffy. We stay with him until then.

He is a truly astonishing person.

—Do you have carers?

—Only twice a day. I like to manage on my own.

—So how do you get from the front room to the bedroom, without the machine? There's quite a long hallway.

—I just hold my breath.

I stare at him.

—*You hold your breath?*

—Yes.

—So what would happen, say, if your wheelchair got jammed in the hallway or you fell out of it or something, when you were between machines?

—I'd die.

He's quite cheerful about it. Val and I stare at him with our jaws on the floor. He looks at our dumbstruck faces and laughs.

—I'm quite independent. I like to do things for myself. Christmas time I had the whole family over and cooked them Christmas dinner.

And the people on *Bake Off* think they have it tough…

We stay with him until the man comes to fix the machine. Then we say goodbye. We tell him to never think he's wasting our time again. Ever.

Jesus. If he only knew.

The list of extraordinary people goes on and on.

Usually 'old' people. The Ukrainian immigrant who saw his family murdered by the Germans, then spent the war down a mine as a slave. The 95-year-old gent, caring for his wife and still sprightly, having spent three and a half years in a Japanese prisoner-of-war camp, eating rice and the occasional snake.

Vince, who – it turns out – is an amateur photographer, interested in Formula One. He's been to the Monaco Grand Prix every single year ever since it began in the 1950s. He's never missed one. As a result, a lot of the marshals have got to know him over the years, and often let him stand to take pictures where they won't even let the professional press photographers stand. As a result he has taken some of the most amazing pictures I've ever seen. There's one of Senna coming down the track in the lead towards Mirabeau which looks like our patient must have been sitting on the car's front wheel. Senna is staring straight at the camera, probably wondering who this maniac is. You can see the whites of his eyes.

Casper, a very pleasant, sprightly American gent, who settled here after the war. He came over with the US forces for D-Day, met a girl, and never went back. Not only that, he was one of the first men onto Omaha Beach on the morning of D-Day. Omaha was the terrible one – *Saving Private Ryan* and all that – and the Americans lost I think over 2,000 dead that day. Far more than any of the other beaches, possibly combined. Our patient was there, and survived. He went on to fight in the Far East, against the Japanese.

Jane, a beautiful lady in her eighties, with long white hair. You can still see how stunning she must have been, all those years ago. She's still stunning now. It turns out during the war she flew Spitfires for the RAF. Later, after the war, she was one of the fastest women on Earth, and the first British woman to break the sound barrier, flying a jet plane.

* * *

All of them sitting up in bed, drinking tea, with me chatting away to them.

And Val rolling her eyes.

—Do you think we could deal with the matter in hand, now?

22

CHILDREN (AGAIN)

It's not just old people who can be amazing. Not by a long chalk. Children can be the worst to deal with.

But also the best.

I started the three-month training course to work on emergency ambulances in 2004. At the end of the first week my head was buzzing with all the lessons we'd had and stuff.

Then Jo said: Oh by the way, I'm pregnant.

Our little girl was born seven months later, the most extraordinary thing ever. It was a difficult, long labour, which ended in a bloodbath even I found shocking, and at one point the midwives thought something was seriously wrong. A doctor came, and tried to work it out. Then it turned out it was OK; she was coming out with one hand over her head, like the Statue of Liberty.

Waving at everyone.

Here I am!

Phoebe

Monday evening. It's just got dark when we're called to a female, eighties, fallen, query injury. This is pretty much the most common sort of call we attend – 'nan-downs'.

There's no key safe at the address and the patient can't get to the door because she's on the floor, so access might be a problem. If we cannot find someone with a key we'll have to get the police out to break the door down. Again, all very routine.

But when we get there a man's waiting for us outside and the front door is wide open. He's an off-duty copper who lives over the road and knows the patient fairly well. We go in to find an elderly lady on the floor who's fallen but is not seriously injured. She has an infection in her urinary tract which is making her very unsteady on her feet, so we decide it would be safest to take her into hospital. We package her up and get her out and comfortable on the ambulance.

—Well if you don't need me any more I'll shoot off, says the copper.

We say thanks a lot and ask him how he got in without a key.

—That was easy. My little girl did it.

—Eh?

Apparently a neighbour had first heard the old lady crying out and had gone to alert the policeman. He'd come across to see how he could help, but neither of them could see how to get in.

So of course what had he done? Went and got a screwdriver and removed the top slit window of the patient's front room, which was slightly open. It's only about two feet across and about a foot deep. There's no chance of any adult getting in through it, even if you could get up there.

Had this been a problem?

Of course not. Now it's time for Wondergirl.

Wondergirl is his six-year-old daughter, who is busy having her tea in his house over the road. She's actually called Phoebe or something.

The copper goes and gets her and takes her over to the patient's house. (Bear in mind it's cold and raining and the house is in complete darkness.) He picks her up and feeds the little girl through the tiny window, lowering her by her arm till she can drop on to the windowsill inside the strange darkened house. Then he lets go. The little girl jumps down into the pitch-dark house and goes off to find the light switches and find the front door and open it to let Dad in.

Fantastic, we think! Where is she?

She's back over the road finishing off her tea.

Well, we can't let the opportunity pass of meeting a superhero, so before we toddle off I go over and knock on the copper's door. Mum comes to the door and I say I want to shake the girl's hand. She is a tiny little blonde thing, tucking into a plate of fish fingers and too shy to come out, so I just say thanks from the doorway. Then it's off to the hospital.

* * *

Another experience I've had as a 'customer' was in 2006. Our daughter was eighteen months old, and Jo was heavily pregnant with our son. One Sunday morning we woke up.

—Shit.

—What?

The bed was soaking. Her waters had broken.

We weren't going to panic. We had a plan. We would drop my daughter off with her aunt, then proceed to the hospital. No problem. But as I struggled to change my daughter's nappy and get her dressed, Jo doubled up in agony. A contraction. Ninety seconds later another one. In other words – birth imminent. Shit.

I called an ambulance.

The crew who came in had had a long Saturday night – this was their last job. Or at least I hope so – they looked dog-rough. So they took her in to hospital. I dropped my daughter off. Our son was born two hours later.

Childbirth.

Simple.

My mother claimed my father insisted on having a paternity test when I was born, just to check I was his, apparently. And when I was going through my mum's drawers when I was a kid, probably looking for money or something, or just bored, I found papers from an adoption agency. I don't know whether it had anything to do with me, but presumably they didn't concern the cat. Later, as a teenager, I had an interview with the army, but was rejected. My father bought me a book about an Englishman joining the Foreign Legion. As if to say: off you go then.

(I'm probably just being oversensitive.)

I often think children are the only really proper thing that's ever happened to me – the only good thing I've ever done.

Jo looks at me like Val sometimes does.

—I think you'll find I did some of the work.

Of course.

23

THE BEST JOB
IN THE WORLD

People sometimes ask how has the service changed you –
what have you 'learnt'? Val laughs.

—What have *you* learnt? Do me a favour.

A rudimentary medical knowledge, maybe, only enough
to turn you into a raging hypochondriac. Headache?
Obviously a stroke. Tummy ache? Probably an aneurysm
that's going to pop. Chest pains? Forget about it.

The answer is I don't know. I've had two children since
joining – everything's changed. I was never really happy
before I had children and joined the service, and I've never
been unhappy since. Make of that what you will.

One day I was walking back from the park with my little
girl. She was three. On a whim I asked:

—Are you enjoying life so far?

She gave it a real think with her three-year-old brain,
pondered it a good long while.

—No.

Oh dear.

Anyway. Life is short and according to the latest medical
evidence, you only get one of them. So make it count.

What does Shakespeare say? *I wasted time, and now doth time waste me.*

(You can see what he means in this job.)

The ambulance service is like everything else: humour goes a long way. George Orwell said to be truly funny, you've got to be serious. He was right. In the service you deal with death and tragedy, injury and illness, misery and loss.

And if you can't laugh about that lot, what the hell can you laugh about?

Another thing you learn – in life and the NHS – is that nothing lasts for ever. Fatima went to another hospital to stare mystified at people after a while, and Len retired soon after this – the years had taken their toll.

And Val and I split up, when I moved to a different area. Last I heard she was thinking of leaving the service.

I miss her.

Frank was the last job we did together.

Frank

It's evening and we get a transfer from the local hospital all the way into London. To the major heart hospital, patient going for bypass surgery. It's an emergency transfer because the patient's condition's serious and the surgeons are waiting, but it's pretty routine for us.

When we wheel the stretcher into the cardiac ward, we find the patient very cheerful, surrounded by his family. The nurses bustle around coolly.

Frank's an affable old boy and very comfortable and stable, no pain, no oxygen, no tubes anywhere. Wife and daughter are there. We get him on to the stretcher, collect the notes and get a quick handover from the nurses, pick up the bags, and off we go.

It doesn't take long to realise the patient's not just affable – he's a lovely old boy. The sort of person who just takes everything as it comes and is a right laugh. He's about eighty or so. Maybe when you get to that age you just don't get frightened. You've had a good life – everything's a bonus. Whatever attitude he's got it's the right one. I hope I have the same. He's enjoying all the attention, joking with us and the staff. If the Grim Reaper does turn up he'll probably sit him down and drink him under the table.

But by the time we get out to the ambulance his daughter's looking morose and his wife's looking worse. She's trembling, eyes staring, white with fear. The surgery he's going for is serious, no question. On his heart, under a general anaesthetic. At his age there's a definite possibility of a bad outcome, or no outcome at all.

The two women watch as we wheel him onto the ambulance and get him comfortable. Now they're both white, and his wife's looking like she might faint any moment. They're asking for directions about how to get to the hospital, slap-bang in the centre of London, through the evening rush hour. They don't have satnav, and they don't have blue lights. They're following up in a car. Maybe they've never even driven into London before.

I can see the fear in the old lady's eyes. She's terrified of the drive, the rush-hour traffic, getting lost, what to do with the car. More to the point, she's terrified this is goodbye. He's going straight into surgery when he gets there, on his heart. At eighty. Maybe she'll never see him alive again. She stands shaking by the ambulance door.

I'm mystified.

—Don't you want to go up with him?

The wife stares at me, speechless. The daughter stares too.

—Can she?

I'm staring at her now.

—Of course. Why ever not?

—The nurses said she couldn't. There wasn't room.

For God's sake, I think. Stupid bastards. (The nurses, I mean.)

—Course there is. Hop on. Make yourself comfortable.

And the wife bursts into tears. She's spent the last three hours – days? weeks? – dreading this one moment, thinking it might be the end. Now she can stay with her husband all the way to the operating theatre. She shins up the steps and into the ambulance. She might yet lose him, but not on our watch. That's good enough for me. That's why I joined the service.

The daughter smiles.

—They said she wasn't allowed on the ambulance!

I smile back.

—Well, it ain't their bleeding ambulance, is it?

ACKNOWLEDGEMENTS

I've had so much help writing this book it's a bit embarrassing. Thanks first and foremost to Frances and Craig, for kicking the whole thing off. To Jane and John and Nick and Gabs for reading it. To Jane at Graham Maw Christie and Lettice and Nicholas at 4th Estate for (practically) writing it. To Jo for putting up with the end of it. And to Sarah and Sam and Cleo and Chris.

Last but by no means least, to colleagues and friends in the NHS emergency ambulance service, the finest bunch of people you could ever hope to meet.